Wheaton Public Library
225 N. Cross
Wheaton, Illinois   60187

A YEAR-LONG NIGHT

Robert Klitzman, M.D.

A YEAR-LONG
NIGHT

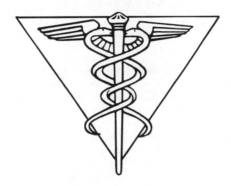

*Tales of a Medical
Internship*

VIKING

VIKING
Published by the Penguin Group
Viking Penguin Inc., 40 West 23rd Street,
New York, New York 10010, U.S.A.
Penguin Books Ltd, 27 Wrights Lane,
London W8 5TZ, England
Penguin Books Australia Ltd, Ringwood,
Victoria, Australia
Penguin Books Canada Ltd, 2801 John Street,
Markham, Ontario, Canada L3R 1B4
Penguin Books (N.Z.) Ltd, 182–190 Wairau Road,
Auckland 10, New Zealand

Penguin Books Ltd, Registered Offices:
Harmondsworth, Middlesex, England

First published in 1989 by Viking Penguin Inc.
Published simultaneously in Canada

1 3 5 7 9 10 8 6 4 2

Although some of the characters in these stories were inspired
by people I have met, in every instance the characters described
are different from any actual person. None of the patients or
hospital staff represent any actual person.

LIBRARY OF CONGRESS CATALOGING IN PUBLICATION DATA
Klitzman, Robert.
A year-long night.
1. Klitzman, Robert. 2. Interns (Medicine)—United
States—Biography. 3. Physician and patient. I. Title.
R154.K37A3 1989 610'.7'1173 [B] 87-40463
ISBN 0-670-81777-5

Printed in the United States of America
Set in Bodoni Book

To my parents

. . . so much of a race depends on how it faces death, and how it stands personal anguish and sickness . . . It seem'd sometimes as if the whole interest of the land, north and south, was one vast central hospital, and all the rest of the affair but flanges.

Walt Whitman, *Specimen Days*

. . . no Greenland winter waits us there,
No year-long night . . .

William Morris, *To Earthly Paradise*

ACKNOWLEDGMENTS

I used to think that the long lists of acknowledgments that appeared in some books seemed excessive. Not until completing this work did I realize how many people are involved.

I would like to thank the doctors, nurses, medical students, and hospital staff with whom I have worked over the last several years. I am particularly indebted to the patients I have seen, for all that I have learned from them.

I also want to thank Dr. Jose Fernandez, Dr. John Sullivan, Dr. Richard Friedman, Matt Wolf, Arthur Chapin, Royce Flippin, and Rob Buchanan for reading drafts of portions of this work, and Dr. Julie Danaher, Dr. Alec Bodkin, Dr. Richard Selzer, Dr. Arnold Cooper, and Warren Stone.

Dr. D. Carleton Gajdusek arranged for me to do research in Papua New Guinea. Dr. Robert Coles provided early enthusiasm and encouragement of my writing.

My thanks to David Leavitt for introducing me to my agent, Kris Dahl, to whom I am especially grateful for her confidence in this undertaking. My editor, Daniel Frank, understood what I was trying to do from the outset and helped guide me there, with his helpful and sensitive suggestions. Finally, Philip Koether offered friendship and support both during my internship and while writing about it.

CONTENTS

II. TRAUMA

III. NEURONS

IV. DEVIATIONS

EPILOGUE

I. Watkins-9

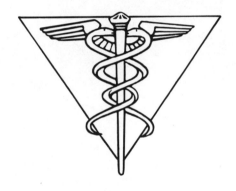

Orientations

"We're very proud of our MICU," Dr. George Barnett announced. He slapped his hand on a square metal box hanging on the yellow wall. A pair of double metal doors swung open with a sigh of air suction pumps as four other new interns and I trod lightly behind him into the Medical Intensive Care Unit.

A hush swallowed us, interrupted only by the electronic beeps of cardiac monitors and the whisper of respirator machines breathing air through light blue plastic tubes beside the eight beds arrayed around the room. The tubes, resembling vacuum cleaner hoses, led into patients' throats and lungs.

Dr. Barnett escorted us over to the first bed on the right. An elderly woman's head was turned to one side. She was unconscious. A nurse was suctioning the patient's respiratory tract with a long plastic tube which she had passed down the woman's throat, and was collecting secretions of mucus clogging her larynx. The nurse let the tube gurgle in the patient's throat, her hand supporting it limply as she watched a television set suspended from the ceiling above the foot of the bed. "The Price Is Right" was playing, and a housewife jumped up and down as the studio audience cheered.

The tube gurgled.

We gathered around the bed. The patient's mattress was filled with specially designed grains of a Styrofoam-like substance that flowed in currents to avoid her developing venous stasis or blood pooling in her limbs, and decubitus ulcers, or bedsores. Short strips of white adhesive cloth tape kept her eyelids closed to prevent her eyes from drying out and to cover her disturbing blank stare.

I was standing near the patient's head, and from around her mouth I smelled a distinctive odor, a warm mix of foul, sour and sweetish scents, like overripe bananas or curdling milk. I had sniffed this heavy scent before. It was produced by the bacteria that flourish in the mouths of the stuporous. I knew this odor from intensive care units I had worked in as a medical student, and associated it with patients who had died shortly afterwards.

I was touring the hospital on the first day of my weeklong orientation to internship. An hour before, I had hurried into the sleek white hospital building and had gotten lost searching for Room 015, the Samuel Lippincott Auditorium.

When I found the room, I joined a cluster of new interns standing around a large metal cart outside the door. Plastic trays supported a huge stainless steel urn of coffee and cardboard boxes of Dunkin' Donuts. We milled around, noisy and nervous.

"Come on now, everybody in!" a short man in a long white coat suddenly called from inside the room. We each grabbed a handful of doughnuts and a Styrofoam cup of coffee, and shuffled into a cool, dark lecture hall. My eyes scanned the rows for a familiar face, or at least a vacant seat.

At the podium stood the short man with the coat. His eyes darted about quickly from behind wire-rimmed glasses as the last of us filed in. He had short-cropped curly hair and a neatly trimmed mustache. "I'm George Barnett, the chief resident," he announced. The chief resident is selected each year by the faculty as the best physician in the class of graduating residents. The recipient of this honor serves as a liaison between the house staff, which consists of interns and residents, and the faculty, training himself in the politics of medicine, arranging schedules and conferences, and defending the department from complaints voiced by the beleaguered house staff. "I want to welcome all of you as PGY-Ones," Dr. Barnett continued. PGY-One means "Post-Graduate Year One," referring to someone who has just finished medical school and has begun internship. "By the end of this year as 'Ones,' " he said, "you will know more clinical medicine than ever again. You'll be different people.

"I want to make a few points. First, you should all have received an orientation packet listing your rotations on different wards, and your on-call schedules.

"Secondly, concerning dress code: I'm not going to tell you how to dress. This was more of a problem a few years ago, I suspect, when some interns wore jeans. Some of the older attendings complained they couldn't tell who were the patients and who were the doctors. Nowadays, just make sure you look like you're here to cure disease, not to spread it.

"Next, I want to mention documentation, and remind you that patients' charts are legal documents. Be careful about what you write. Also, not all abbreviations are accepted. A book of acceptable and unacceptable abbreviations is included in your packet.

"And finally, I want to tell you about my first night on call as an intern. I had just met twenty-four patients that morning and hadn't yet gotten to know any of them or much about them.

The emergency room called to say that a patient there was about to be admitted to my service. My first admission had landed on the floor an hour earlier, and I hadn't even eyeballed her yet. Meanwhile, one of the patients on the ward was having chest pain, another was spiking a temperature. A few minutes later, I got my third hit of the night." He referred to new patients as "hits." He neither joked nor apologized. The corners of his mouth strained downwards, his eyes focused in a permanent scowl, anticipating disaster.

I was excited but afraid. Would I relish the chance to tackle catastrophe as he evidently did? I glanced around. We interns were all stiffly uniformed in "whites," as the white suits of jackets and pants, or skirts for the women, were dubbed. We had all just finished medical school and had slaved to be accepted by this prestigious teaching hospital. As medical students we had read textbooks and thought we knew what we were doing. Internship would test us.

"You can't save them all," Barnett told us, "but you can sure learn." When no more could be done to help the sick, interns would continue to work for the sake of education. I was reminded of my orientation to medical school four years earlier. The Dean had sobered us, saying, "Students enter medical school wanting to do good. They leave hoping to do well."

I flipped through Xeroxed handouts jammed into my newly purchased clipboard, frantically trying to memorize the complex map of hospital wings and buildings. Some wings bore two names, others three. The Morgan Pavilion was also known as the G wing. Letters, numbers, and names swirled like alphabet soup. I thumbed through computer printouts of intern assignments, on-call schedules, rules, regulations, and accepted vocabulary, resembling the laws and language of a foreign country. Internship was divided into a number of rotations on different wards. The first half of my year would be spent on a general medical ward, Watkins-9, after which I would rotate through neurology and pediatric wards, and work in the Emergency Room as well.

Dr. Barnett finished his tale and was replaced at the podium by the Engineering Department representative, who was wearing a short-sleeved white shirt and a drab chocolate brown tie. He was without a white coat. "I want to welcome all of you," he grumbled into the microphone. "We want you all to phone us for any problems. If any piece of hospital furniture or equipment is broken, if you spot a blackout or a flood in a hallway, don't assume someone else has already called." He rapidly spun off other possible disasters. To him, the hospital was a place where machines broke down and got repaired.

The hospital attorney, a tall man in a gray suit and black glasses, followed. Rearranging and perusing the papers on the podium before him, he said, "I can't overemphasize the importance of what your own Dr. Barnett has told you about documentation. You must be careful nowadays." He looked up as if establishing eye contact with a jury. "Anything you write in a chart may be used for or against you. Your licenses can be revoked if you're not careful. In recent lawsuits, an intern or resident who errs, even on one case in the emergency room at three in the morning, can be indicted, his state license jeopardized and possibly lost. Also, don't make the chart a battleground. If you disagree with someone on a case—a resident, a fellow, a consultant, or an attending—talk to them about it. Whatever you do, don't let these arguments spill over into the chart, which may be read by lawyers, the government, and insurance companies. Dispute spells bad news. Your safest bet is to document everything about a patient. That way, you won't neglect anything. If you act in good faith clinically, you'll be acting in good faith legally as well. And if a lawyer contacts you about a case, call us before you talk."

A psychiatrist then spent twenty minutes advising us on how to ward off stress. He passed out copies of an article that reviewed research on the subject. "I personally like to read the scientific literature about problems like this," he confessed. "I frequently use intellectualization as a defense mechanism. I think it's a good one."

With that, we drifted out into the hallway, where we formed teams for tours of the institution. My leader happened to be Dr. Barnett.

"Okay, is everyone here?" he asked as we flocked together in front of him. He didn't count, and none of us knew. "All right, let's do it." He bustled down the corridor as if running an emergency blood sample to the lab to save someone's life.

"What wards are you all starting out on?" Dr. Barnett asked us.

"Morgan-10-G-10-South, the cancer ward," a woman in front of me, Erica Chin, volunteered. She spewed out the syllables in a single breathless phrase. Her black hair, cut just above her shoulders, swayed as her short legs raced to keep up with Barnett's pace.

"Oh, it's great there!" Dr. Barnett told her. "Everybody's real sick. It's like one big intensive care unit.

"How about you?" he asked looking toward me, part of a group that had begun to lag behind the expedition.

"Me?" I asked. "Watkins-9." I already envisioned myself galloping up and down nine flights of stairs throughout the day and night.

"Some say it's the Plaza up there, but you'll see great pathology," he told me. By "great pathology" I knew from medical school that he meant obscure maladies: pheochromocytomas, insulinomas, multiple myelomas. "Fascinomas" they were dubbed, exotic but classic diseases, rarely seen but prized because they could be definitively diagnosed by specialized laboratory tests when suspected. Their existence confirmed that medicine could be scientific.

As we trotted down the hallway, the page operator suddenly coughed on the overhead speaker. *Paging Dr. Spencer, 4803, 4803. Paging Dr. Faust, 8310, 8310.* Instinctively I strained to hear. The fuzzy syllables were pushed through the staticky sieve of a speaker. Hospital extension numbers dropped out of the sky. I had been conditioned to struggle to catch them.

The page operator called out the physician's name only once but repeated twice the extension number he was to contact in response. The doctor's name was often in doubt. In one of the hospitals where I'd worked as a medical student, Dr. Schutzman and Dr. Klitzman were always responding to each other's names. "Dr. . . . zzzman" was often all I heard clearly enunciated. Anxiety bloomed when I thought I heard my name called. Was that me? What was that number again? Who wants me? Will it be a call that takes thirty seconds to respond to, or a problem that will claim me for the rest of the night?

Paging the Television Hostess, stat. 7025, 7025.

Attention please. Attention please. The flower arranging class is now beginning in the L-Nine conference room.

Men strode by in suits, children sprinted down the hall ahead of their mothers, a white-haired man propelled a wheelchair. People talked of where they wanted to have lunch. This corridor might have been at an airport or subway station. The page operator reminded us that this was a house of the sick.

We followed Dr. Barnett down the hall and halted behind him at the double doors. "This is our last stop on the tour," he announced. "The Medical Intensive Care Unit."

I had been in hospitals before, training in them as a medical student. But the final year of that long educational process is spent less in these institutions than in outpatient clinics and advisors' offices. During the series of lectures in the morning, internship had still seemed far off—someone else's hell. The sounds of the corridor had jarred me into recognition. But it was in the MICU—seeing and smelling a stuporous patient—that the world of the hospital once more engulfed me. Medical school had sheltered me behind textbooks, but her stench and her decaying skin now pushed themselves upon me.

My internship had begun.

Admissions

On the day after orientation, I hurried toward the hospital. As I neared the building, increasing numbers of people on the sidewalk were dressed in white. I passed the medical center bookstore, where a window displayed new textbooks, a skull, a complete skeleton, and plastic models of an eyeball, an ear, and a fetus. Across the street were three florist shops, their windows filled with bright flowers.

I came to the hospital's circular driveway, bustling with taxis, buses and vans. Elderly people tottered through the revolving doors at the entrance or were being rolled out in wheelchairs. Younger family members carried vases, pots of flowers, and valises. They kept to the sidewalk while I cut across the drive.

My first destination was the security office, Room 024, in the sub-sub-basement, to pick up an ID badge. The freight elevator I rode opened onto a hallway where dulled fluorescent lights flickered from the ceiling. Pieces of equipment lay stranded against the yellow tiled walls—crippled hospital beds with missing wheels, office desks without legs, wheelchairs with cracked axles or ripped backs, and battered filing cabinets. A wheeled stretcher had lost its mattress, and had become a metal table. Rows of lockers were banked against the wall, used by the electricians, kitchen workers, and janitors who made the hospital run. Men hauled long dollies, piled with boxes and equipment. I passed the boiler room and the hospital laundry, where bales of sheets and uniforms, stained with blood, iodine, and urine, were piled, waiting to be tumbled into huge washing machines.

At the security office, I lined up behind other interns as an obese guard slowly snapped our pictures and laminated them onto cards. He plodded along at his own pace, deaf to our protests about being made late on our first day.

Finally, a glossy photo was clipped to my white lapel. The snapshot had caught me smiling awkwardly. I entered a sleek and shiny passenger elevator and rode up to my new home—Watkins-9.

When we stopped at the first floor, a crowd of people packed into the car. Two nurses in white skirts stood beside me. An older nurse with steel gray hair entered the elevator behind them and kept her distance, nodding her chin a few millimeters to acknowledge them. A tight white paper hat only three inches wide was pinned to her bun, indicating that she was a head nurse. It was no more than a parody of a hat. By now, nurse's caps have pretty well disappeared. The few one sees are holdovers from the past, worn usually by older nurses who cling to this symbol of status.

On the fourth floor, a kitchen staff employee entered. Miss Steel Hair still stared directly ahead, silent and aloof. With patients and staff sharing elevators, doctors and nurses are often reminded to keep their tongues still. But occasionally staff people will chat about a patient, heedless of the possibility that their subject's family may be standing beside them. Lawyers trying malpractice cases have reportedly donned white coats and eavesdropped on conversations in hospital elevators, overhearing otherwise unobtainable information about a case.

Finally, the elevator reached the ninth floor, and I made my way toward the center of my ward, Watkins-9, to find the nursing station. At a reception desk behind a glass panel sat a woman in a navy blue smock.

"I'm one of the new interns," I said, introducing myself through the round opening in the glass.

"Uh-huh, I'm Mathilda," she answered, not looking up from the papers on her blotter. She appeared to be in her early forties. The hospital insignia was sewn to her smock and her name was embroidered in script above her breast pocket.

"What's your code?" she asked.

"My what?"

"Your code. Every doctor has one. It's a five-digit combo of letters and numbers that gets written on all your patients' lab slips. You'd better call the house staff office today and find out what your code is, because you're going to need it."

"Thanks," I said, surprised by this greeting. I walked past Mathilda's desk into the station. The nursing station was the closest thing to a staff lounge and was the central brain of the complex organism of the ward. On one wall stretched a bulletin board where various documents were posted. A multi-page memo was entitled "Hospital Disaster Plan." On the bottom of the sheet was the notation "To replace previous disaster plan, memo #3021-R." Also on the corkboard were thumbtacked postcards from distant places presumably sent by patients long gone. There was also a small placard: "Reduce Entropy: Put Away Your Charts."

In one corner of the nursing station a coffee machine dribbled rich brown liquid into a Pyrex pot. A sign above it requested donations of twenty-five cents per cup to be placed into an empty tin can. On a dusty windowsill, a small geranium squatted in a foil-wrapped pot on which a piece of paper was taped. "Please water me," it read, "or I will die."

At the end of the room, a small group of doctors was gathered. Four house officers were stationed on each floor: three interns and—as their immediate supervisor—one resident.

"I'm Walt Simmons," a tall man in his mid-thirties said as he thrust his palm toward me. A wide tie, fashionable in the late sixties, was loosened around his neck, the top button of his shirt unfastened. He had black curly hair. "You must be a rookie like me," he said. He tapped out a cigarette from a pack of Marlboros, lit it, and set it down in the plastic lid from a Styrofoam cup of coffee.

"Is it that obvious?"

"I can see the water behind your ears." He laughed and inhaled on his cigarette. His glasses were held together at one corner by surgical tape. A medical student I'd known regularly used surgical tape to adhere his glasses to his nose so they wouldn't fall off. Once, when he was peering over a patient during an operation, the spectacles had dropped and bounced onto the sterilized skin.

A woman sat cross-legged in a swivel chair next to Walt, her short white skirt and white coat telling me she was an intern too. "I'm Joan deMonzo," she said, as we shook hands. A mass of curls tumbled across her head and down one side. Her red polished fingertips snipped off pieces of a large chocolate chip cookie as she sipped a diet Coke through a straw.

A man in a white coat flipping through a stack of index cards beside her held out his hand. "Emmanuel Velos, your resident. Welcome," he said, smiling, his eyes warm. He was slim and compact, and fine featured except for his large, almost floppy ears. His curly hair was cut short. Two black fountain pens were clipped in his breast pocket.

"Which one of you is on call tonight?" he asked us.

"I am," Joan answered. "I like diving right in. I'll get to know my patients better." She had already folded up the sleeves of her white coat. Four or five bracelets encircled her wrist.

"We're probably going to be here late every day this week anyway," Walt said.

I agreed. If a patient develops a problem after five o'clock, his intern, if still in the building, is responsible for handling the situation. If the intern has already left for the day, the work falls to the DOC, the Doctor on Call. The longer an intern hangs around, the more problems accumulate to detain him.

"I'm not looking forward to this," Walt said. "As an intern— a scut monkey—the only people who're going to respect us are the medical students." "Scut" described the chores an intern has to do for his patients.

"I don't mind," Joan confessed. "I've been waiting for a long time for this . . . since high school. We've finally made it. I figured my life wouldn't really start until I got out of med school. I was a real nerd," she said, giggling. "I'll probably end up marrying a doctor, too."

"How come?" I asked.

"It'll be easier. I won't have to explain every night when I come home late what I spent my day doing."

"Are you dating a doctor now?" Walt asked.

"No. But I've decided that's what I want. In the old days, doctors used to marry nurses all the time. I once thought about becoming a nurse."

"Really?" Walt asked.

"Yes. But for all the bother, I thought I might as well go to medical school."

"I don't blame you. Nurses don't always get respect, anyway. Some nurses are wonderful, but they vary. You can often save a patient from pneumonia but you can't always save them from some nurses."

"What do you mean?"

"They'll come up to a doctor and say something like, 'Excuse me, I think Mrs. Humphrey just exploded,' " he mocked in a falsetto.

"Was anyone in your family a doctor?" Joan asked.

Emmanuel answered the question. "My dad is."

"What kind?"

"A general practitioner. He's a family doctor in a small town. He has a nice practice. Neighbors seek him out for advice on everything—whether to get a divorce, quit a job, which college to attend, whether to go to medical school. It's not a bad life."

"Is that what you want to do?"

"No. But it has influenced me in a lot of ways. I prefer treatments that are 'low tech.' " He explained that he was skeptical of the technical overkill of hospitals with their expensive tests, and instead valued thoughtful clinical judgment. He seemed like he would be kind and attentive to patients' feelings.

"What are you thinking of specializing in?" Joan asked him.

"Endocrine. I want to stay in academic medicine and teach. What about you?"

"I'm thinking of Derm," Joan answered.

"The skin team, huh?" Walt commented. "You know the three laws of dermatology?" She looked at him, puzzled. "If it's wet, dry it. If it's dry, wet it. And whatever you do, don't touch it." He laughed.

"You'll get a taste of most subspecialties during internship," Emmanuel pointed out.

"How did you find the year?" Walt asked him.

"Long. Long hours plus plenty of paperwork. You'll spend a lot of time here in this station, filling out forms, composing notes and telephoning, serving as your own secretary."

"Are you glad it's behind you?" he asked.

"Sure. It's important not to let the job get to you too much. There are a few things you should remember. First, never eat hospital cafeteria food. It's depressing. When you're on call, the Department of Medicine usually supplies dinner. If they don't, order out for delivery. We usually got Chinese food or pizza. When I was depressed, I'd splurge and order out for sushi. Also, you have to keep the rest of your life going, or you'll just die. I tried to go jogging twice a week and played squash. You should try to go out every night after being on call, even if it's to a movie and you just fall asleep from having been up all night. Sometimes, I just went to the local diner. . . .

"But time's running on," he said, looking at his watch. "We should start rounds. Here are sign-out sheets describing your patients, written by the interns who just finished." He distributed a piece of paper to each of us. "You each have eight to ten cases. Why don't we see them all briefly together. Then each of you can go back and spend more time with your own patients individually."

The first person we saw, Mrs. Rutherton, had been assigned to Joan. We listened to Mrs. Rutherton's heart thump in our stethoscopes and her lungs whisper like seashells reporting the sound of distant disease, the extent of organ damage. Our four stethoscope bulbs danced over her back, jumping to different spots after each of her breaths. We listened to check if there were any wheezes, rubs, rales, gallops, or murmurs, sounds that are potentially dangerous and easy to hear.

We traveled from one patient to the next, inspecting sites of disease and surgical incisions. I was most interested in the patients that were to be mine, but we saw them all. Walt began to look tired. "You know what I call rounds?" he whispered to me wryly. "Shifting dullness." This is a medical term used to describe abnormal fluid that moves about in a patient's abdomen when he rolls on his side. The belly sounds dull when tapped like a drum, indicating the presence of liquid—pus or protein leaked by damaged tissue.

When rounds were over, I prepared to go back to visit each of my new patients, alone. I had trouble imagining this ward as my new home. Like the patients, I was just passing through, playing doctor, acting the role, and making up the script as I went along.

Did I look the part of the physician? I didn't want the patients to know that this was my first day, and wondered what they were feeling about being assigned a new doctor.

I wandered out to meet the first one.

Miss Steiner's Room

I left the nursing station and entered the first room on the right. I consulted my list of patients.

"Good morning, Miss Steiner," I called out. "I'm to be your new doctor."

"Wonderful," a guttural voice answered flatly. I knew from the sign-out sheet and from Emmanuel that Victoria Steiner was an eighty-one-year-old spinster, never hospitalized before, who had been brought in because of a broken arm. Congestive heart failure and withering kidneys had been discovered. She was deaf in her right ear and partially deaf in her left one. When I walked in now, her head, topped by tousled white hair, lay propped on a pillow. A light blue plastic oxygen mask the size of her entire face had slipped, and now hung loosely around her neck, blowing cold foggy gas onto her chin.

"Miss Steiner, your mask fell off."

"Yeah, yeah," she snapped. She waved a frail hand in the air as if to say, "Look, I don't care, just leave me alone."

19

I repositioned her mask, and shouted into her less deaf ear, "How are you doing, Miss Steiner?"

"I'm doing, I'm doing." Her eyes stared at the ceiling, ignoring me.

Her private duty nurse, a svelte black woman in a crisp white uniform, interrupted her. "Miss Steiner, you have to tell the doctor what's going on with you." The nurse sat on a chair at an angle beside the head of the bed. On her lap was a tabloid newspaper, her finger hooked between the pages, holding her place.

"Yeah, yeah, I'm telling, I'm telling." The nurse gave me an exasperated look. "I'm wonderful," Miss Steiner said.

The nurse, whose badge said 'Ruby Parsons,' smiled at me. "She's not taking her medications, doctor."

"Why aren't you taking them, Miss Steiner?"

"Because I don't want to."

With heart failure, her lungs could drown in their own secretions. Drugs were needed.

"She isn't drinking either, doctor."

"Are you drinking?"

"Yeah, yeah, I'm drinking."

"All she does is take sips."

"Miss Steiner, if you don't drink and don't take your medications you won't get better."

"So?" she answered.

"Miss Steiner, do you want to get better?"

"No."

"Miss Steiner, do you want to die?"

I couldn't believe this question had slipped out of my mouth.

But from beneath her mask she muttered, "So, I die."

Her tiny body lay beneath the sheet, naked but for white gym socks on her feet. Her mask hissed and puffed, spewing white clouds all around her. She looked like some octogenarian astronaut, ready for take-off from planet earth.

Three feet away, at right angles to Miss Steiner's bed, was another, in which sat Mrs. Harriet Knocks, a fifty-five-year-old woman with metastatic lung cancer. A plastic curtain separating their beds was drawn to one side.

"How are you, Mrs. Knocks?" I approached her bed.

"Fine, fine," she said in a raspy voice. She was wearing a wig and was busy applying makeup. I assumed that her hair had fallen out during a previous course of chemotherapy. She put her eyeliner pencil down beside an assortment of bottles and boxes lined up in front of her. "Pretty busy morning with my friend over there, huh?"

"Not bad."

"She pulls that every day. Don't let it bother you. I can tell she likes you. She's a sweetie underneath." She lifted a cigarette from an ashtray on her nighttable and took a puff.

"How are *you* doing today?" I asked.

"Me? I'm fine." She took a drag on her cigarette, then squashed the butt in her ashtray. It was eight in the morning, and she was battling lung cancer. I glanced down into her overflowing ashtray. "You must think I'm crazy," she said, "still smoking. I am crazy, aren't I? But what can you do?" She laughed. "I can't quit. Even with this. I can't bring myself to stop."

There was no point reminding her that smoking causes carcinoma of the lung. Cigarettes were one of the few pleasures she had left, an old habit. Like her roommate, she was testing limits, undermining efforts to help her. I could pump as much chemotherapy into her body as it tolerated, but she would continue to smoke.

While I listened to her heart and lungs, she called out to her roommate, "Victoria, you be nice to our new doctor, you hear?" Miss Steiner's mask nodded. "She'll be good," Mrs. Knocks promised in a gruff whisper, winking at me. "I'll make sure."

"Doctor," Ruby said as I started to leave the room, "you know Miss Steiner refused blood drawing this morning." The hospital phlebotomist makes his rounds at 7:00 A.M. in order to speed the specimens to laboratories as early as possible. Testing takes hours.

"Why did you refuse?" I asked Miss Steiner.

"Because."

I would have to sample her blood myself. I bustled off to the supply room across the hall, in which were lined metal supply carts equipped with drawers of tongue blades, Band-Aids, toothbrushes, razors, kits for spinal taps, and other essentials. I collected what I needed—a handful of alcohol pads, squares of cotton gauze, a needle, and three empty glass tubes with rubber stoppers.

Miss Steiner's right arm was strapped in a sling, and her left arm was bruised from dozens of previous punctures that had mottled it with hematomas—purple splotches from burst blood vessels. I peeled off the paper backing on a plastic package containing a butterfly needle. A plastic tube was attached to two orange wings that folded upwards perpendicular to the needle itself, allowing my fingers to guide the attack. Behind these orange flaps, a long cord twisted, which I inserted into a hollow socket called a vacutainer. The socket would receive the sealed test tubes into which her blood would be drawn. I tied off the blood return from her left arm with a tourniquet. A single vein coursed between two purple patches, but it wiggled as I poked it with a needle and then it popped. Blood leaked out to form another hematoma. I loosened the tourniquet and clamped a square of cotton gauze down on the site with my thumb for three minutes. Miss Steiner continued to stare at the overhead light. I hurried back to the supply room to fetch a new needle.

This time I tied the arm farther toward her hand, below the

new hematoma, and tried another spot. My brow was sweating. The next vein also ballooned out from oozing blood. Mrs. Knocks observed the whole scene and rolled her eyes with amusement. I held down the vein and squeezed it harder, trying vainly to stop the leakage of blood. Several times I ran back to the nursing station, first for more gauze, then for another needle, then for additional alcohol wipes. Walt, my fellow intern, leaned against a counter near the supply room, chatting with an attractive nurse.

"Looks like bad news," he joked when he saw me replenishing my supplies. "She's a hard stick, huh? Watch out for these 'hema-tomatoes.' " When I passed him a second time, he shook his head. "Tough luck, man. When you've got a patient with multi-system failure, you've got a long day ahead of you."

My heart raced. Was I going to be this slow at everything that had to be done?

Finally, I gave up on the left arm and switched to the arm with the sling, more difficult since I wouldn't be able to reposition it. But I hit a vein square on and the blood flowed.

I swore to stock up on supplies by stuffing the pockets of my white coat and to stay calm.

I ran back to the nursing station. "I need this sent off," I told Mathilda, the ward clerk.

Mathilda grumbled. "Just leave it right there. I'll get to it."

That wouldn't do. "It has to be sent off 'stat.' " Which means urgently. I needed the results by that afternoon.

"Stat," she said and smirked. "That's the only word you doctors seem to know around here." I knew from being a medical student that the normal pace of a hospital often wasn't fast enough. But no doubt many things were labeled "stat" to move them along.

"You'd better fill out the slips yourself then," she said.

"Where are they kept?"

"Back there," she said, pointing to a row of shelves behind her desk. I squatted down to hunt among the slots for various-sized forms.

"But don't you go taking all of mine," she added. "And don't you forget to put away the charts you use, you hear?" she threatened. "Because I don't want to be cleaning up after all of you. Interns can't find anything the first few days. I have to whip you all into shape."

I found and filled out the request slip. "Excuse me," I said. "How does it get sent down?"

"Don't look at me," she said, not lifting her eyes from her blotter where she was filling out a form of her own. "You call the escort service and they'll come up when they can." My list of chores was growing.

An employee from the escort office happened to be standing in the hallway, about to deliver a patient to Radiology, not far from the lab.

"Do you think he would mind bringing it down for me?" I asked Mathilda.

"You can ask him," she told me, "but I doubt it. That's not in his job description."

It was on his way, though, and he agreed to deliver the blood sample for me.

I was relieved that at least one chore was completed.

The next day, I detected the hint of a faint smile behind Victoria's mask and a sparkle in her eye. "You look cheery today, Miss Steiner."

"Yeah, yeah. I'm cheery, I'm cheery." Still, she refused to grace me with a smile or glance.

I approached Mrs. Knocks's bedside. She was sitting up, preening herself before a mirror, brushing her wig. A telephone receiver was hooked between her cheek and her shoulder. "It's Harriet . . ." she was saying. "I'm fine. I'm in a semiprivate room. The other woman's very sick. Oops, the doctor's here. I have to go. I'll call you back later, dear."

I'd learned that only recently had she informed friends that she was in the hospital. At first, she had wanted to keep it a secret. The only family she had was an estranged daughter who had moved to California and contacted her mother rarely. Harriet's husband had died of a heart attack twelve years earlier. She didn't want to bother her friends with her problems, she'd told one of the nurses. But eventually she had informed them and now chatted on the phone regularly.

I had brought syringes of thick polished glass, loaded with chemotherapy: clear fluids, the bright purple and orange colors of varieties of Hawaiian Punch, and sticky, like syrup. For a number of my patients on the ward I injected chemicals that would "lyse," or disintegrate, tumors but would kill normal cells too. The potions were measured by fine calibrations delicately etched into the glass. A dozen chemicals were blended in various combinations for use as chemotherapy against different cancers. The mixes were known by their acronyms: MOPP (an abbreviation for nitrogen mustard, oncovin, procarbazine and prednisone), CHOPP, COPP, and BLAM.

One of Mrs. Knocks's chemicals was packaged in a plastic bag and had to be dripped through her IV tubing slowly over an hour. I hung the sack from her IV pole and connected it to a machine that would slowly pump the fluid. A red sticker on the sack showed a skull and crossbones printed in bold black ink with the legend DANGER—POISON.

"Is this stuff going to kill me or what, doc?" she asked sardonically.

"It's supposed to help."

"You're gonna cure me with magic, huh?"

"It's been shown to work in many cases."

"Maybe I can take a bath in it." She tapped her pack of Winstons and pinned a fresh cigarette between her lips. "So, doc, I saw a great movie on TV last night," she chatted as my fingers eased a glass plunger into a polished syringe, past black lines ticking off volume.

"What was it?"

"An old Fred Astaire–Ginger Rogers number. I guess they're before your time, huh?"

"They're classic."

"Let me tell you, if I had it to do over, I might've been an actress. I have the voice, don't I?" Her voice crackled like an old record, warm and rich but hoarse.

"Maybe." I wasn't sure if its resonance rose from her vocal cords or resulted from her cancer.

She suddenly waved, peering over my shoulder as two friends walked into the room. An elderly man in a gray suit and homburg hat hobbled behind his wife, who bustled up to Mrs. Knocks and kissed her pale and pancaked cheek. "Have you met my doctor?" Mrs. Knocks asked. She introduced us, and they smiled and shook my hand.

"Why don't you go say hello to Victoria over there?" Mrs. Knocks suggested to them. "She's all alone and has no one." They ventured across the room where Victoria's oxygen mask was covering her ear as she stared upwards. "How are you?" Mildred asked very slowly.

"All right."

"She's such a dear," Mildred uttered in a loud aside to her husband. "You take care now."

Victoria elevated her hand an inch or two off the bed to wave, granting more of a response than I had ever earned.

Once every week or two, Miss Steiner's only visitor came

by, a niece who lived in an expensive area of town not far from the hospital. "Can I bring her in some food from outside?" the niece asked me one day. "I think she'd eat more if she liked the food better. I know a great macrobiotic Oriental vegetarian restaurant near me. Don't worry, they don't use any salt or MSG. They make great stir-fried vegetables." She ordered out for delivery from a pay phone in the hallway. But Miss Steiner didn't consume any more of it than she did hospital food.

As a private duty nurse, Ruby was hired to care for only one patient. A floor nurse, Diane, ministered to ten or fifteen patients and was forced to rely on her own common sense to answer questions that arose. "Diane, can you check over these medication sheets I've written out?" Ruby would ask. One patient was easier than fifteen. But Ruby was new to hospital routine and obsessed with details.

"I'm too busy now. Later sometime," Diane would answer. She had to supervise Ruby's work, but avoided her questions, out of lack of time and jealousy of Ruby's less arduous assignment.

Ruby had time to buttonhole me and lobby for Miss Steiner's interests. "Can't I give her her diuretic with her other meds? Can you change the order? It'll only take a minute." She would page me to ask whether Miss Steiner should receive her bedtime meds at nine or at ten.

I often had more pressing errands to do but I would grant Ruby's requests. She earned my sympathy. I commiserated with her having to tolerate Miss Steiner's wrath.

Ruby wore the purest white dresses of any nurse. Miss Steiner had her share of stains, but Ruby kept her wardrobe pristine and Miss Steiner's room immaculate. She never voiced complaints about Miss Steiner. That wasn't her place, though she had her views. Her boyfriend, Clyde, was a technician in the chemistry lab, and occasionally visited her on the floor. They'd retreat to my on-call room, a small chamber with a cot where I slept when on call. I tried not to disturb them.

With only one patient, Ruby was often bored. She usually read magazines in her chair by Miss Steiner's head, and chatted with Mrs. Knocks.

"Could I ask you a favor?" Mrs. Knocks would ask her. "Could you go get the paper?" When I entered their room, the pages of a newspaper would be spread out between them on the bed. It was the only way I got to see what was going on in the world. "Gorby Says 'No,'" the banner would read. "Aide Attacked," the front page would declare one day; "Aide Resigns," the next. These headlines constituted the outside world for me. During internship, I rarely had time to watch TV, listen to the radio, or peruse the paper myself.

I looked forward to stopping by "Miss Steiner's room," as I began to call it. Patients whose care was more routine blended together. I brought less of myself into their management, administering the standard doses of medicine and care. Mrs. Knocks treated me with annoyance, if not disdain, and smoked fiendishly, defying her cancer and chemotherapy. Her feisty cynicism sustained her. Still, it was Miss Steiner with whom I battled the most, a *grande dame* around whom everything revolved. I had to work hard to convince her to let me help her.

One morning after I had known her for about two weeks, Miss Steiner's breathing grew more labored. Fluid pooled in her lungs. The amount of oxygen stored in her blood dwindled, and Ruby, Diane, and I hoisted her onto a stretcher to be transferred to the intensive care unit. "Let's go already," she mumbled.

Off she went, rolled down the hall surrounded by Emmanuel pumping an oxygen bag, Diane holding a sack of IV fluid up in the air, and me steering the rickety stretcher with her chart tucked under my arm. Her mask hissed as she stared upwards, ignoring us. Ruby remained behind in the room, collecting Miss Steiner's few possessions.

A few hours later, I was sitting in the nursing station when a sharp *ding* startled me. "Yes, may I help you?" Mathilda answered, speaking into the patient intercom.

"Yes, darling," I heard Mrs. Knocks's voice through the static. "Could you get me a glass of water, please?"

"Just you wait, I'll tell the nurse." Ten minutes later, the intercom rang again. "Where's that water?" Mrs. Knocks snapped. "This is the second time I've had to ask."

That night on call, I spotted Mrs. Knocks stationed in the hallway, which was unusual. She waved hello with her fuming cigarette. She had posted herself on a bench by the elevator, the only seat in the hallway. I suspected she wanted to escape being alone with her illness. Anyone who came on or off the floor that night passed her by. "Are you here all the time?" she asked me. "You poor thing. Don't you ever sleep?" It was among the most sympathetic comments I ever received during my year of nights in the hospital.

"Do you want the patient in nine-eleven to get a sleeping pill?" Rita, the night nurse, asked me a few hours later.

"Which patient is in that room, again?"

"I don't know."

"Well, can you check?" She then scanned an erasable board of names and room numbers posted at the nursing station.

"Knocks."

"Okay."

Doctors almost never know patients' room numbers, only their names; interns and residents stay on a ward for an average of only one month. But it's the other way around with nurses, who remain there for years, assigned part of a floor, Rooms 908 to 914, for example, and identify patients by those numbers.

I followed particular patients, the ones I had admitted when on call and the ones handed down to me by my predecessor. I divided my work up by individual patients and thought in terms of a disease acting itself out in someone's body. I followed the progress of Mrs. Knocks's tumor, knowing that her room was the first one on the right. The rooms themselves seemed identical in my mind. What distinguished them were the patients inside. I recalled Mrs. Knocks's disease, the sound of her lungs, the texture of her skin.

"How are you doing?" I asked Mrs. Knocks the next morning in the now half-empty room. She was probing her breakfast with a metal fork on a tray before her.

"Badly."

"Why is that?"

"I can't stand these eggs," she told me. "They usually give you a piece of bacon with it and you can shove it down."

I hadn't eaten breakfast at all.

"Could you sit up so I can listen to your lungs for a moment?"

"Anything to get away from those eggs. What do you want me to do?" She seemed distracted.

"Just breathe in and out through your mouth as usual," I said, placing my stethoscope on her back.

"How's she doing?" she asked, interrupting my exam. She didn't bother to point over to Miss Steiner's empty bed. We both knew whom she meant.

"She's stabilized," I said, meaning she wasn't getting any worse. Often it's the most positive comment I can make about a patient's status.

"I don't know how she did it," Mrs. Knocks mused. "If I were her, I'd be scared out of my wits. She was such a frail thing, a real doll, though, wasn't she? Even when she gave you a hard time."

The next day, Mrs. Knocks was sitting in Ruby's old chair,

pulled over to the edge of her mattress, her arms folded and propped up on the bed, her forehead nestled into their comfort. Her face was hidden. It looked as if she were bent down before an altar.

"Mrs. Knocks?"

"Oh, it's you, honey," she said, looking up.

"Good morning."

"I got the shake and bake from the chemo this morning," she said and sighed, referring to the trembling rigors and the fever that often accompany administration of the medicine. "I haven't gotten nauseous or sick yet from it, though. I must be some kind of freak of nature." She hadn't applied her makeup. Her wig sagged on a Styrofoam mannequin's head beside her. She was too ill to be self-conscious about her baldness.

Over the next several days, she stayed secluded in her room while I came and left each day. "Things here just aren't the same," she muttered. "You're so busy these days." I had other rooms to go to, more patients to see. What I saw was how they each struggled to piece together some shreds of defiance and dignity in a world that was falling away.

Dr. Barnett, the chief resident, stopped me in the hall the next day. "I'm looking for good patient material; you know—good teaching cases to present to medical students. Do you have anything?"

I repeated the phrase to myself: "Good patient material." I thought of Mrs. Knocks and how she felt about her illness. She was a good patient. But "good patient material"?

I wasn't sure if this attention would help her or be seen as an intrusion, but I gave him her name.

"Thank you for sending those lovely students in to see me," she said later. "They're so young. They asked all about me, though."

"Thank *you*. I'm glad you didn't mind."

"I must be an interesting case, huh? A model patient." We smiled.

Mrs. Knocks completed her treatment one week later and went home to return in a month for more.

A few days later I was hurrying through the hospital lobby.

"Remember me?" a young woman with curly brown hair called out. "Miss Steiner's niece."

"Oh yes," I said. "How did she do?"

"She went down to the unit. Then she was put on another floor. I was there every day with her, her only visitor. Well, she eventually died." She paused. "Her last words to me were, 'I don't need you anymore.' "

"That's too bad," I said.

Her niece shrugged. "That's the way she always was."

Long after that, I continued to call it "Miss Steiner's old room."

IVs

"Judy, I'm going to have to put an IV in your neck."

"No way."

"But no veins are left in your arms or legs."

"I said no."

"The fluid is essential."

"Don't I have a choice?"

I pondered for a moment. "You do, but it would be medically foolish."

Judy Langdon had been admitted to the hospital three days earlier, after fending off abdominal and ovarian cancer for nine of her thirty-three years. Her private attending physician, Samuel Ross, had followed her from the beginning. He was an aging but suave man with cavernous eyes and silver hair brushed across the top of an expansive forehead. He didn't spend much time with interns, though I was to be responsible for Judy's day-to-day care. "I spoke to your resident about the case already," he told me when she was admitted. "I don't have time to repeat everything. Why don't you talk to him first?"

Judy Langdon had outlived her doctor's forecast. He evaded discussing her prognosis anymore. She had consistently disproved him. Her belly was bloated from tumors obstructing her intestines. The growths bulged in her lungs and studded her liver and pelvic structures. A tube punctured her right flank and snaked toward her kidney to rechannel her urine; a bag glued to the front of her abdomen rerouted her colon. Now with her intestines again clogged, she had ceased drinking and had dried out.

Her small head lay beyond the rising mountain of her stomach, as if she were pregnant. When I had lifted away her hospital gown to examine her, my hands felt the hard bulges of tumor floating on the surface of her intestines, wobbling beneath a thin tissue of flesh. Her skin, pulled tautly over these bulges, was quilted with healed incision lines from countless surgical procedures.

On her first night, she had required a nasogastric—or "NG"—tube to evacuate her stomach.

"Lean your head forward, please," I had requested. A slender coil greased with Surgilube K-Y jelly dangled before her.

"Nice deep breaths now; it'll be finished soon." She complied and the pipe slid down her throat, encountering resistance at various points, which the thrust of my gloved hand overcame. Liters of muddy, green-brown fluid poured out, easing tension that had built up in her abdomen for weeks. She also needed hydration through an IV, and on her pale arms I located the faint streak of a single hair-width vein. After two days of these two conduits, the dehydration resolved. But she wasn't healthy enough to go home.

The IV was needed to supply her with medications and ample water to prevent dehydration. She didn't take anything by mouth. The catheter tunneled from the dirty external world, through her protective coat of skin, into her sterile bloodstream. It had to be changed every three days to avoid becoming infected. Bacteria might easily penetrate this gap in her body's defenses.

On the third night, I again knotted a tourniquet around her upper arm. She automatically pumped her bony hand, coaxing her veins to stand up. I poked, prodded, and kneaded her arm, but this time, no veins rose to her skin's surface. They had all collapsed or exploded from the multiple lines that had been started over the months and years. They had retreated or been spent. I moved around her, strapping and searching each limb without luck. There was only one recourse.

"Why *don't* you want the line in your neck?" I asked, exasperated.

"It's gross."

"Why?"

"It'll make a scar." She might live only for a few more months. Still, her protests were a sign that she was improved from her acute crisis of sudden blockage. She was returning to her chronic state of slowly succumbing to the disease. Medical science draws a critical distinction between acute and chronic problems, those that demand immediate intervention and those that go on for months or years, with physicians incapable of reversing the onward push of gradual deterioration.

"But, Judy, it'll only be a tiny, faint line, maybe nothing at all."

"I don't want it."

"We don't have a choice!"

"I don't believe this," she whimpered.

"I'm sorry." My arms folded.

"It's so unfair." I didn't budge. Tears moistened her eyes. "I suppose . . . If you must."

A nurse, Rita, stood by my side, handing me supplies as I pierced Judy's neck with a needle, aiming toward the middle.

"Ouch!" Judy winced.

"I'm sorry," I said. I didn't like inflicting pain.

"Relax, honey," Rita told her in a gruff voice.

"One more millimeter," I was thinking. I could accidentally puncture her lung if I probed too deeply. My brow tensed and perspired. "Be careful," Walt had warned me right before I started this procedure. "I've never popped a lung. But you have to be careful." His words were haunting.

"One degree over to the right," I reflected, "and I should be in her internal jugular." Blood dripped from the hole, smearing like watery paint.

"Is this necessary?"

"Let the doctor here do what he has to do." Rita's support surprised me, as she was usually cool or antagonistic toward me.

Finally, through the curls of tubing a line of blood looped like a roller coaster. The vein had been lanced. I taped the tubing to her thin skin. "There, it's all done. That wasn't so bad, was it?"

The next morning, Judy pouted. "Do you know this is the longest time I've ever gone without looking in the mirror?" Her wide brown eyes glowed warmly.

"Is that right?" I sensed a rebuke.

"Almost a whole week." She blinked. Her illness had made her facial features even more delicate than they must have once been.

"Why is that?"

"Because I can't make it to the bathroom anymore. Can you imagine that? Me not looking into the mirror a zillion times a day like I've being doing since high school? It's amazing.

"I had a dream last night," she continued, "that I would live happily ever after. I was surprised."

"Why?"

"I haven't lived very happily up to now."

By her bedside glowed expensive lavender packages from a boutique. On the side shone the stylishly printed word "Obsession."

"What's 'Obsession'?" I asked.

"It's a fragrance by Calvin Klein." The product had only just come on the market. Dressed in loose bed sheets with four tubes outfitting her body, this emaciated woman connected herself with the outside world by something as ephemeral as a fragrance. She couldn't bring herself to have food, but she had "Obsession." Her husband, a successful businessman, had brought it to her. He visited only once a week, taking a taxi from downtown, and was dressed in an expensive suit, a starched white shirt and a silk tie. He invariably brought gifts.

They lived in an elegant chrome-and-glass apartment building, which I occasionally passed after work. On each floor, sliding doors led out to sunny terraces. I'd wonder which apartment was theirs, curious about her life off the ward. I knew some of her secrets—the scars that marked her body, the extent of tumors pressing her organs, her blood counts—though others were inaccessible. I didn't know her fantasies, how she relaxed at home or decorated her living room. Before becoming ill, Judy had been a successful commodities trader, managing money and clients. Now, she managed her illness and negotiated with me. Nine years ago, she and her husband had vacationed for the summer in Italy and had picked out and purchased a villa as a second home. That autumn, she became sick and was stamped with her diagnosis. Her life since had revolved around the hospital.

"Any problems today?"

"My throat's scratchy. Could you give me something for it?" Cooped up in the hospital, she had developed a mild sore throat and a cough.

"How about an antiseptic spray?"

"Will it get rid of the irritation?"

"Let's try it and see."

The next morning her first words to me were "It didn't do *any*thing."

"What didn't?"

"That spray stuff you gave me yesterday. Can't I get something stronger—with codeine?"

I hesitated. Should I prescribe a potentially addicting medication? I checked with Emmanuel. "Sure, give it to her," he answered nonchalantly. "Maybe it'll help." Admittedly, the quantity of codeine in the cough syrup was small.

"Why is it," she asked the next day, "that every time I come to the hospital for bowel obstruction, some other problem becomes more important? Last time it was anemia, this time my throat." She gazed beyond my shoulder as she asked. The problems she chose to focus on were the small ones that could be solved.

Each day after visiting Judy, I ventured into the adjacent room, occupied by Mrs. Kunoshi Nakamoto, a slender Japanese woman with metastatic lung cancer. She was born and raised in rural Japan, and after World War II, she had come to the United States and met her husband, whose family was from the same province as hers. She'd worked hard and raised a daughter and a son. Two years ago, her cough had begun. For months she'd refused to see doctors, and drank a special herbal tea sent to her from relatives back in Japan. But the cough never left. "She's dying," Emmanuel had warned me on my first day. "Don't spend your time with the dead."

"How are things today?" I asked her.

"Not fresh," she uttered, condemning a grapefruit sitting on her tray. In her dim, simply furnished room, she was wearing a beautiful silk kimono. The sun streamed into her dark chamber and illuminated the silken skin of her cheek. The grapefruit glistened on the thin table before her.

"Anything else?"

"Short of breath." This was an ongoing problem. Cancer riddled her body and there was little more we could do for her.

"I'm going to remove the IV, Mrs. Nakamoto."

"No, don't take it out! The IV makes me better."

"But you're drinking enough liquid by mouth, so you don't need it, and an IV can become infected." Salt water alone dripped through her line.

"No, you gave me an IV when I was sick. The IV keeps me alive." Her right hand reached tremulously for the piping, which wound toward her left arm. She grasped the hollow plastic as if to protect it from my approach.

I backed off.

IVs are not what they seem. A former patient once recollected that the most memorable event of her hospitalization was me removing her line, cutting off the white cloth tape that had secured it to her arm. After two and one-half weeks of IVs, she felt unshackled. Other patients experience this removal as a loss: diminished nurturance, nutrients, and hope. The agitated and angry yank their lines out themselves, and even demented patients otherwise oblivious to their environment sense what's tying them down. Their arms worm free in the most energetic and coordinated set of movements their bodies can muster.

As I left Mrs. Nakamoto's room, Jennifer caught up with me in the hallway. "Judy Langdon wants to speak with you." Jennifer was a stout nurse with plain features and a heap of chestnut hair piled atop her head. A loose yellow and green soccer shirt hung rumpled on her body along with baggy white pants. Her white clogs were streaked with black scuff marks.

"But I just saw Judy."

"She says she forgot to ask you something."

I walked back to Judy's room. "What's up?"

"I want to eat." She still had an IV and an NG.

"You may not be ready for that yet." Fluid had stopped draining from her stomach, but appetite usually takes longer to return.

"Can't I try?"

I admired her determination. "All right, I'll pull the tube and we'll see how you do."

"When?"

"Probably later today, when I get a chance."

As the day unfolded, though, new admissions and a few emergencies claimed my time. Judy's tube had been in place for several days and I assigned it lower priority on the list of tasks to be done.

Jennifer paged me. "Judy keeps asking when you'll remove the IV."

"As soon as I get a chance. I'm in the middle of an emergency," I answered.

A few hours elapsed before I arrived to free her. I untaped the tube from her nose and withdrew it from her esophagus. A film of green grease coated the plastic. "Get that thing out of here," she exclaimed.

I ordered her a light breakfast.

But in the morning, she scrunched up her nose. "Euh," she exclaimed. "They gave me some disgusting cereal with milk. How do you expect me to eat when you give me that crap? What do you think I am, anyway? Some kind of garbage dumpster?" I ordered a more advanced meal but she barely picked at it.

Her body began to lose what little weight it had managed to maintain, and she required larger volumes of fluid. She was switched to total parental nutrition, or TPN—IV feedings of protein, glucose, fats, and vitamins essential to functioning.

Individual formulas were prepared daily for all TPN patients, depending on measurements of the salts and chemicals in their blood the previous day. This complex preparation of chemicals was recorded in the order book and was more akin to medication than food.

"Is this going to help me?"

"It should. It's filled with nutritional requirements."

"I like it already." Nothing else could be offered.

In the next room, Mrs. Nakamoto continued to deteriorate. She was still conscious but grew drowsier, sleeping longer each day. As I came by each morning, she'd just nod to my questions without opening her eyes as I warmed her hand with mine.

How long a patient survives is often determined by his or her "code status." If a patient has a cardiac or respiratory arrest—if the heart stops or breathing fails—emergency measures can be undertaken to attempt to resuscitate the patient. A hospital-wide code can be called, with physicians from all over the hospital galloping in, summoned by the page operator. "Code Six," she would chant in order not to alarm other patients, and she would add the location of the arrest. A doctor runs to "a code" where a patient "is coding." At a hospital where I worked as a medical student, the house staff was divided into "arrest teams." The page operator would call, for example, "Team A," followed by a location. The house staff would say that a patient had "teamed."

Some hospitals have floor-wide codes in which some but not all efforts are made, with only some of the possible people involved, employing a limited number of the conceivable medications and machines. The staff may respond with deliberate slowness, too. Finally, a patient might be allowed to die in peace, with orders written in advance that state "Do Not Resuscitate." They die naturally, without any attempt to prolong the process.

Arrangements for code status and for autopsies must be made with the patient and his family. The attending physician is officially responsible, but this task, as with most, often falls to the intern. Some patients were DNR on a previous admission but weren't now, either because they were healthier or because the beleaguered house officer hadn't arranged with the attending and the family to make it official. It was time to discuss Mrs. Nakamoto's code status with her family.

I met with her husband, who didn't speak English, and their only daughter. "We may not be able to do much more for your mother," I warned her daughter, who dutifully translated into Japanese. Mr. Nakamoto nodded.

"We like to talk about this with families because problems may arise in which we have to make a quick decision whether to take special measures to keep a patient alive."

Her daughter's thin lips squeezed together. She turned to her father and translated the message. He peered down at his lap and uttered back something in Japanese. "My father says he understands. He knows that you have tried hard to help." He looked into my eyes with sad trust.

"We would like to arrange that if she should suddenly become more dangerously ill, we will make her comfortable, but not take heroic measures that may require machines to breathe for her."

"I understand," she answered.

Mrs. Nakamoto was made "DNR." The order was written: "In the event of cardiopulmonary arrest, Do Not Resuscitate."

A few days later, Judy became sicker. I ordered X-rays to be done and went down to the Radiology Department to obtain the results.

The radiologist, Dr. Flint, was gazing at a large X-ray on an illuminated screen. "Did you see Langdon's films?" I said, interrupting him.

"They're over there," he announced, pointing with his elbow toward a pile of X-rays without glancing over.

"What'd you think of them?" I ventured to ask.

"Lots of mets"—"mets" are metastases, or colonies of cancer. "She's dead," he said casually. He pulled the X-ray from his viewing box and slipped another one in its place. He had never seen Judy. I shrank away, dropping her pictures into a manila envelope. Their plastic edges scraped along the rough paper and they clunked to the bottom.

Judy told me her thirty-fourth birthday was coming up, just four days away, on the following Monday. I wasn't sure she'd make it. But four days later, to the surprise of the staff, she was still alive. At the last minute, Jennifer ordered a cake from the hospital kitchen for her. It arrived on the floor along with the morning shipment of medications. All day, it sat on a desk in the nurse's station, yet no one had the heart or the courage to bring it in to her.

Finally, late that afternoon, I said, "Why is this still sitting here?"

"Because it's sad," Jennifer explained. "She won't be able to eat it."

"But it's her birthday," I protested. "What else can we do? Stick a candle into her IV bottle?"

"Do you want to be the one to bring it in to her?"

"Okay. But let's all do it together." Seven of us marched in—the ward clerk, Mathilda, and the floor janitor, Greg, plus Emmanuel, Walt, Joan, Jennifer, and me.

"Happy Birthday to you," we sang. We sang the song all the way through, and then clapped. Judy managed a slight smile, and we stood in awkward silence. Jennifer massaged Judy's bony hand. "Maybe you can try tasting a little bit of the cake," I said.

"Whatever you don't eat, we'll help you with," Emmanuel blurted out. It was going to be the last birthday cake she'd ever have—probably the last food she'd ever eat. She shook her head with her little remaining energy, declining even a morsel. After a minute, Jennifer cut the cake and passed it around to us on paper towels. We ate it hungrily, without a word, glancing at Judy from time to time, who looked down at her rounded abdomen and occasionally up at her IV pole. We each drifted out of the room when we finished our serving.

The next day, Jennifer paged me. "The patient in Room Nine-o-nine is in a lot of pain."

I walked into the room and saw immediately that Mrs. Nakamoto's torment had increased. I started her on a drip of Levo-dromoran, an opiate similar to morphine. This powerful drug would numb her body and brain, dropping a veil between her and the external world. She didn't comprehend my explanations and warnings that it was a mind-altering substance, and a desperate measure. When "Levo," as it's called, is begun, the end is near. I could do nothing more to help than ease her unrelenting agony with around-the-clock opiate. I ordered the drug for her as if it were sugar water.

A short while later, I ducked into Mrs. Nakamoto's room again. The drip hadn't yet been hung up. Out in the corridor I ran into Jennifer. "What happened?"

"I got upset when I went in there. She's in such distress."

I barely managed to hold my temper. "Do it now," I said sharply, and she hurried off.

Mrs. Nakamoto continued to look worse.

Her breathing accelerated, and more concentrated oxygen was sprayed through her mask.

I tinkered with these two essentials—oxygen and pain-killer—increasing the rate of the drip, titrating between the amount needed to quell pain and the quantity that would put her to sleep.

The next morning, Mathilda paged me on the intercom. "Jennifer wants to see you—now!" The firmness of her message communicated its urgency. I rushed.

Jennifer met me in the hallway. "She just expired."

"Who?"

"Mrs. Nakamoto. You have to pronounce the body."

I walked into the room, somber. The patient lay completely still. Eight family members were crowded together in the shadows around her bed, where they had huddled since the previous afternoon. Mr. Nakamoto sat in the front chair, alone, nearest his wife, watching her as if expecting something to happen. I'd never "pronounced" someone in front of an audience before. They knew what had occurred. I glanced over at her IV, still dripping. In a small oblong collecting bag at the top of the tubing, the salt water swelled into droplets that fell one after another.

I took my stethoscope from my pocket and listened to her heart. The only sound was her moist skin sticking to the plastic bell. Was her heart shifting faintly? No. I pressed the bell on her chest. Again, nothing. Looking up at her calm face, I could almost see her still breathing.

To declare her dead legally, a note in her chart would have to state that in examining her I'd found no breathing, no heartbeat, and no response. She looked unarousable, but I had to know for sure. It seemed to me that my signature, which would officially pronounce her dead, had never carried such irrevocable weight. Grasping her shoulder and rocking it gently, I raised my voice a little. "Mrs. Nakamoto?" I was presuming to wake the dead. "Mrs. Nakamoto?"

The family was waiting. They all knew my findings.

I lowered her shoulder onto the bed. "She's dead."

I let her go.

The family members nodded their heads, relieved.

An hour later, they left. Her body was wrapped in a plastic sheet and quietly wheeled down the hall to the rear service elevators. When I was a medical student, my first sight of the day each morning as I climbed the five steps from the parking lot onto the loading dock of the hospital had been a row of six-foot-long black boxes being rolled out from the freight elevators into the icy daylight. Few things in a hospital are painted pitch black. A special forklift lowered one box at a time into the back of a waiting station wagon.

Mrs. Nakamoto was one of the first patients I had cared for who had died. Could I have done more to help her? Emmanuel assured me, no. Death is an accepted, often expected outcome.

Judy never knew of Mrs. Nakamoto. She was preoccupied by her own condition, which continued to worsen after her birthday. Her weight stabilized but her body ached.

"I want to leave here," she said and sighed one evening when I was in her room. Her husband happened to be seated at her bedside.

"But you need to continue getting fluids through your intravenous line," I pointed out.

"I want to go home."

"Judy, you'll be out of here soon," Mr. Langdon urged.

"But home is life to me, and the hospital is illness. I want to go home, away from this, to my own home."

"Don't give up now," he beseeched her.

"I've already lived twice as long as I should have with my diagnosis. I'm a survivor. I should have been dead years ago. I know what it is that I want."

I admitted that it might be possible for her to have an IV at home, if we could arrange a private duty nurse to care for it.

"But I don't want an IV."

"You need it," her husband insisted.

"All along, throughout this whole thing, I've always thought of the hospital as being the place with all this junk," she said, waving her hand at the portable blood pressure meter and the forest of IV poles towering above her as she lay on the bed. "I want to go home. With nothing."

"But what's an IV?" her husband objected. After all that she had been through, he didn't want her to die from dehydration.

"IVs are part of the hospital. They don't belong at home."

"It's just fluid."

"It's more than that."

Her husband's head dropped into his palms.

"Would you let me come home without it?" she asked him.

His head shook heavily in his hands.

She sighed. "Then I guess it can come home too."

There was still an obstacle, however: persuading Dr. Ross that it was all right for her to leave. He had seen her brush against death before. Though incorrect about her prognosis, he had come to be proud of her. And himself. He had invested years of time into her care, overseeing years of crises and near misses.

"Dr. Ross," I said to him in the nursing station, "Judy Langdon has been asking me if we can send her home, since there's nothing we can do for her here."

"Nonsense. What is she going to do at home? She still needs to be here in the hospital."

"But she probably doesn't have long to live."

"You don't know her the way I do. I've seen her through this before—worse than this. You'll see. No, she's staying here."

"But we could maintain her IV at home."

"I've made up my mind. I'm not giving her up now—not yet."

When Judy learned of this, she called him at home that night. "Please, Dr. Ross," she pleaded. "It's all that matters to me."

"We've pulled you through bad times before, we'll see you through this one too."

"But I want to go home now. I don't want to be here anymore."

A few more days passed in which this battle waged, as she and I tried convincing Dr. Ross to recognize the situation. Meanwhile, Judy steadily deteriorated. She developed a fever, and though we started her on antibiotics, her temperature continued to soar. Blood, urine, and sputum cultures revealed no source of infection, and her chest X-ray ruled out pneumonia. Raging tumor was the culprit.

"Maybe we can't do much else for her," Dr. Ross finally admitted, gazing at the temperature graph in her chart. "She can go home if she wants—but with an IV. Stop her TPN. Blood tests would have to be drawn daily to monitor it, and she doesn't want them done." Dr. Ross rose and walked away.

Several more days were required to institute the necessary plans, to move oxygen supplies and IV bottles into her apartment, and to hire and instruct a private duty nurse. She would receive only basic IV fluid—salt water and a little glucose. But this blend would be as transparent as plain water, and she would notice that her fluid had changed from yellow to clear. She'd wonder why, and fear that Dr. Ross and I had given up. Dr. Ross decided to add vitamins that colored the bottle the same bright shade of yellow it had been before.

While the arrangements were being made, Judy's condition became more tenuous. Her pain escalated. "Dr. Ross, don't you think we should make Judy Langdon DNR?"

"That's premature."

"It looks like she's slipping downhill."

"At some point, yes, maybe we can discuss it. I'll have to sit down with her husband first. I don't have time for that now."

"But Dr. Ross—"

"Not now. Let's just keep her status quo."

When Mr. Langdon visited the next evening, he asked me how I thought Judy was doing.

"Not well, I'm sorry to say."

"I know. Her time's running out. I don't want anything special done to help her, you know. Nor does she." He and I had been contemplating the identical problem. I spoke with Dr. Ross again, and he finally agreed. Do Not Resuscitate orders were written.

The next evening, Mr. Langdon brought her a diamond ring. He placed it on her night table, but she was too weak to reach it. Holding her frail hand up, he slipped it on her finger, and held her in his arms as she wept.

Nothing could tame her pain now but opiates, and she was started on a Levo drip. Her alertness now faded to drowsiness and stupor, whether from medication, carcinoma, or both.

I phoned the visiting nurse service several times to speed up the arrangements for her return home. Finally, late one afternoon, a nurse was assigned and supplies were in place.

"So long, Judy," I said, clutching her hand. "Good luck."

"Thank you," she whispered, only half awake. Unfortunately, as an intern, I saw patients only when they were in the hospital. Once they left, I might never see them again, and would often never even hear about how they fared.

With the discharge order written, she was rolled down the hall out of her room toward the elevator bank. She hadn't left her room in weeks. Behind her trailed nurses carrying vases of roses and carnations, packages from boutiques, and a menagerie of stuffed animals she'd had with her, which had increased in number as she had become sicker. Her husband didn't come to escort her home.

I walked along behind the procession. The stretcher was wheeled onto the elevator and her companions squeezed in alongside, holding her belongings above her. She was not fully aware that she was being discharged. I stepped back into the hallway. The automatic doors clamped shut.

Devo Chemo

The day Howard Kirby was diagnosed with leukemia, he arrived home in a brand-new Buick. He was a reserved fifty-eight-year-old accountant who had risen slowly through his corporation and was not ordinarily given to flights of caprice. One week later, he was to receive his first round of chemotherapy.

This first hospitalization proceeded smoothly. Unfortunately, subsequent tests showed that the medicine had failed to arrest his cancer. A few months later, he was infused with a second barrage. He was readmitted to the hospital now by his attending physician, Dr. Karl Rohr, to learn if this second treatment had worked.

His wife and three daughters were assembled around his bed when I walked into his room. "Hello, I'm Dr. Klitzman, the intern who'll be helping to take care of you."

"He has hemorrhoids, you know," his wife said. "You better put him on Colace."

Need for a stool softener seemed the least of his problems. However—"Thank you for telling me that," I said soothingly,

and asked questions about his leukemia: when it was diagnosed, what his symptoms were, what treatment he had received. I had learned to bypass the patient's immediate com-
plaint if it was unrelated to his major illness. His hemorrhoids
weren't discussed further.

That night, Dr. Rohr arrived on the floor, tall, tanned, and
athletic-looking. In contrast to interns and residents, whose
coats were jacket length, his white coat reached to his knees.
A former chief resident, he still worked long hours. He kept
a large framed photograph of his wife and two children on the
desk in his office though I heard that he rarely saw them.

Dr. Rohr performed a bone marrow biopsy, inserting a thick
needle into Mr. Kirby's pelvic bone and quickly withdrawing
it. The specimen was sent to the pathology lab to be read.
"It'll probably take a day or so for the result," he told us. The
contents of this narrow core would predict Mr. Kirby's fate.

The next day, the results were ready. Dr. Rohr wasn't around
and it became my job to transmit the findings.

"I'm afraid I have bad news for you, Mr. Kirby. The results
are back. Your marrow still contains leukemic cells." His
marrow was "blasting off," exploding with premature blood
cells, known as "blasts," from his leukemia.

His pale face became even whiter. "The second set of treatments didn't work?"

"They didn't."

His glance fell into his lap. He was sitting up in bed, visibly
shaken. His family was collected around him, his wife sitting
rigidly on a light blue vinyl easy chair, gripping its arm rests.
One of his three daughters slumped in a desk chair, her feet
stretched out before her. Another daughter had hoisted herself
up onto the windowsill and squatted on the radiator grill, staring
at the gray floor. The third sat cross-legged on the ground,
Indian style, crying.

"Are you sure?" one of his daughters asked.

"That's what the pathology report says. I realize this is very upsetting."

"Is there nothing else that can help me?"

"Maybe experimental chemotherapy. It's not guaranteed, you know. But it may work."

Dr. Rohr was affiliated with the Department of Developmental Chemotherapy. Later that day, I returned to Mr. Kirby's room accompanied by Dr. Rohr. "We can try you on HHT-AMSA, a new experimental chemotherapy," Dr. Rohr told them. This blend of chemicals was being explored as a treatment for leukemia with some initial evidence that it might work for certain patients. The potion, made from the bark of a tree that grew in China, was rumored to be so potent that when some of it once spilled on the floor, it burned a hole in the tiling.

"I think we should do it," Mrs. Kirby announced.

"What's it involve?" asked Mr. Kirby meekly.

"There's a long list of side effects I can give you," Dr. Rohr said. They included malaise, nausea and mucositis, high blood sugar, low blood pressure, fluid retention, liver dysfunction, and cardiac arrhythmias.

"Can we think about it?"

"Take a week. Then let me know your decision. I wouldn't postpone it any longer than that if I were you." Mr. Kirby could face the natural course of his illness or be a guinea pig for a new and not fully tested "protocol" of medications. A newfangled drug could attempt to forestall fate. Dr. Rohr performed an about-face and retreated from the room, leaving me to make any necessary arrangements for the discharge.

"You're not on any medications, right?" I inquired. "So you don't need any prescriptions."

"Well, could you give Valium?" his wife asked me.

"Why is that?" I could imagine the reason, but I needed to

hear a patient's problem from him or her directly before prescribing drugs, especially ones that were potentially addicting.

"Because of what we've been through today," his wife said angrily, "what we found out." Here was a dying man. I pondered whether to prescribe a drug that might not be strictly needed. Should I be more concerned with easing his suffering than with avoiding possible habituation?

I asked Emmanuel.

"He's no doubt under a lot of stress. Sure, you can give him some."

I returned to my patient. "Okay, I'll give you a week's worth."

"No," the daughter sitting on the floor interjected. "We all want Valium!"

"All of us need it," Mrs. Kirby added.

I gazed down at her and then at each family member. They looked distraught. But they were not my patients.

I reconsulted with my resident. "They all want Valium?" Emmanuel repeated, surprised and amused. "Just give him some extras," he said, not concerned with the particulars. Writing prescriptions was easy from his perspective. Valium was a ubiquitous medication which many internists prescribed regularly for anxious patients. It was one of the most commonly ordered drugs in all of medicine.

Compared with some other medications, Valium's side effects were few, though over months it could become addicting. I was troubled providing it to a family I didn't know and might never see again. But Emmanuel knew the practice of prescribing medications better than I did at this point, as well as the value of expeditiously discharging a patient—in this case a whole family.

I handed Mr. Kirby a generous prescription.

At the time I didn't consider whether I'd opt for the experimental treatments if I were in Mr. Kirby's place. I didn't imagine myself as ever being a patient.

A week later I saw Mr. Kirby back on the ward. I went into his room to gather an updated history and perform a physical exam. We had been through an ordeal together, and were friends of sorts. "You were in accounting, I understand," I said conversationally as I wrapped the blood pressure cuff around his arm.

"Was?" he remarked, startled. "I still am." He paused. "You'll be here for the next four weeks, won't you?" he asked.

"Yes, why?"

"Because that's how long I'm going to be here. Longer than the two other chemo trials that failed me." Perhaps he believed that because the treatment was longer, it was more likely to succeed. "They told me that even with this, though, I only have a thirty-percent chance of being saved." His bluntness astonished me; he spoke as if he had just four weeks left of life.

"How many minutes before I get my medicine?"

"Three hours."

"Can you let me know when it'll be ten minutes before?"

"Why is that?"

"I just want to prepare."

At 1:50, I alerted him. His wife was with him.

"Do you really think I should go through with this, doctor?" he asked.

It was late for second-guessing himself. "It's your decision."

"Honey, what do you think?" he implored his wife.

"Let's do it," she answered, impatient with so much discussion.

He sighed his agreement and nodded. I returned, hung the bag of medicine up to his IV pole, and threaded the plastic tubing through an electronic pump that pulsed with drops of the chemical. I screwed an attachment onto his IV line and took his pulse. "What's my heart rate?"

"Ninety-two."

"Isn't that abnormally high?"

"Anxiety can increase it. Try to relax."

"Can you list all of the side effects again?"

"Seriously?"

"Please." I wondered if refreshing his memory about the symptoms would lead him to imagining he suffered them, but I repeated the list.

Over the next two days, Mr. Kirby did well. Hope helped make him better. When, a few days later, he became mildly nauseous, this side effect was treated.

Each day, developmental chemotherapists in long white coats flocked into the nursing station behind Dr. Rohr and surrounded me. "On Mr. Kirby . . ." Dr. Rohr would start, "I want his blood counts checked twice a day, and watch his weight, he's not eating." Such were the commands I was ordered to follow. Dr. Rohr flipped open the patient's chart, uncapped his pen, and scribbled a brief, illegible note, signing it, "Devo Chemo," for Developmental Chemotherapy.

Emmanuel later sat down and read aloud to me what had been written. " 'Patient has no shoes today.' "

"No shoes?"

"Yes, that's what it says."

"You sure it doesn't say 'was nauseous'?"

"That may be what they meant, but what they wrote was 'no shoes.' "

I spied over his shoulder. He was right.

Through the course of internship, my own writing had deteriorated as well. My signature shrank from my full first and last name, to my first initial and last name, then to my initials followed by a bumpy squiggle representing the letters of my last name slurred together.

Mr. Kirby became septic a few days later. Bacteria invaded his bloodstream. The chemo slowly racked his body and he grew weak and febrile. He looked wan, his hair thinned, his cheeks caved in, and he started vomiting several times a day. The drug was largely responsible.

"Do you have any questions?" I asked him one morning on rounds.

"Just one," he answered. "When does one cross the line from merely being weak to dying?"

Who could answer this question? Whatever line he imagined as existing, we both knew he was in the middle of crossing it.

"I don't know," I told him sadly.

Mr. Kirby worsened progressively. "Make me better," he pleaded one morning. "Do anything you can."

"What do you mean?"

"I have had enough." Wrinkled pale blue pajamas clung to his sweaty flesh. Loosely scattered about his skull, his hair looked about to slip out.

"Howard, the medicine may help you," his wife urged.

"Mona, I feel wretched."

"That'll pass, though. Isn't that right, doctor?"

"Hopefully, yes."

"Howard, we've tried everything else. You know what it was like being sick at home. That was worse."

"This is awful."

"You tell him, doctor," she said, turning to me. His family and Devo Chemo backed the medicine. The patient was opposed. To whom would I be loyal?

"The medicine may be very rough. In the end, you're the only one who experiences that, Mr. Kirby. It's your decision."

"What do I do?"

"You'll have to speak to Dr. Rohr."

At least some of his suffering might be relieved by ending this effort to help him. "First do no harm," I had been taught in medical school. If he had a cardiac or pulmonary arrest while on the experimental protocol, a code would be called.

While he was receiving this medication, his status couldn't be changed to "Do Not Resuscitate." As long as he continued to participate in the research, he couldn't be rescued from whatever extraordinary measures Dr. Rohr would take to save him, including, for example, a respirator machine. He had signed over his life to his attending physician.

"My husband's in agony," his wife told Dr. Rohr in the hallway that afternoon.

"The medicine might soon begin to take effect," Rohr argued.

"But he's suffering so!"

"We're already this far along," he told her. "He's had six of the twelve treatments. Why don't we wait a little longer?"

"Can't you speed it up or do anything else to help him?"

"He might turn around any day now."

"He's begging me to have it stopped."

"Don't you want to try to help him?"

She sighed, defeated. "I guess we can wait for now."

During the days that followed, Mr. Kirby's skin yellowed like paper as he became jaundiced from cholestasis, or bile backing up because his liver was too diseased to metabolize it. "What do you think?" his wife asked me one day.

"I think it's up to your husband and yourself. You should do what you feel is right."

"Can't you just stop it?"

"It's not up to me, I'm afraid." In the nursing station, I spoke to Rohr myself. "What do you make of the Kirby case?"

"Hard to say."

"Do you think the chemo will help him?"

"I don't know. We're still trying it out. There have been individual case reports that it has worked. But it may take years to know for sure." He didn't want to lose his research subject. He wanted to find out whether his concoction worked. Research studies require research subjects.

"Would you consider stopping it on medical grounds at any point?"

"Possibly. It depends."

"On what? What would that point be?"

"I suppose if he developed a ventricular arrhythmia we'd hold it"—that is, if the heart's ventricle beat at its own erratic pace, uncontrolled by the usual electrical pathways. Even that might only be temporary.

"He is experiencing other side effects, though. Do you think we should consider at least interrupting the protocol before that happens?"

"Let's wait and see."

"But he's suffering."

"His vital signs are still stable. His electrocardiogram hasn't changed."

"So we're just going to keep giving it to him?"

"For now. We'll continue to follow him closely." Dr. Rohr shut the patient's chart and recapped his pen. He walked away, leaving me standing alone.

I next saw Dr. Rohr in the medical library, where we interns regularly gathered for a lunchtime lecture. The discussions were usually on topics like "Subtypes of Thyroid Cancer" or "Treatment of Testicular Carcinoma." This day, we met with several senior residents and attendings to discuss our experiences thus far at the hospital.

First Emmanuel treated us to sound advice. "No matter how hard you try," he said, "no matter how much good and correct work you do for patients, they may still get very sick, they still may die."

Then Dr. Rohr spoke. "Often in oncology, a treatment becomes standard because we have nothing else to offer patients. We have some treatments that work very well for some cancers, but for other kinds of tumors, we are less successful.

"The drugs we offer can be dangerous, and often more toxic

than our patients' diseases. Many people are killed by their therapy here, rather than by their illness. It can be disturbing."

I left the meeting disheartened. I had thought that Mr. Kirby's predicament was unique, but it was not.

That afternoon, Mr. Kirby's pulse became irregular: the arrhythmia Dr. Rohr had described earlier had developed.

"Mona, you have to do something," Mr. Kirby urged.

"But this is the last hope the doctors think they can offer you."

"It's been too much already."

"But if you don't get this, there's nothing else."

"I know, but I want it stopped."

"Are you sure, Howard?"

"That's all I wish for now."

"Doctor, we've decided," she told me. "We've had enough."

"I understand, but you should speak to Dr. Rohr about that."

Later that day, she told Rohr, "You have to stop it."

"Are you refusing the treatment?"

"I am," Howard spoke up. His comments had become sparser in recent days.

"All right then," Dr. Rohr said. "Good luck."

Rohr told me in the nursing station, "Recheck his EKG. Then you can discharge him when he's stable."

"Just like that?"

"That's what I said." Rohr seemed indifferent. The chemo was halted, and his pulse returned to normal, but Mr. Kirby never fully recovered from its other effects. Finally, though, he went home.

His last morning, I entered his room on rounds to say goodbye. It was already empty. "Where's Mr. Kirby?" I asked the nurse.

"He left."

His bed stripped, his night table bare of his few possessions, it was as if he had already died.

Another Player

"Trick or treat?"

I was walking down the ward briskly one morning when Edward Rainer stopped me. It was Halloween time, and swinging alongside his IV pole as he rattled it up and down the corridor was a plastic orange pumpkin. He wore a white mask, plain and featureless with holes cut out for his eyes. From one end of the hall to the other he strolled in green socks, offering candy. He had decorated the IV stand, taping on flowers, some plastic and some real. Artificial roses bloomed from green plastic stems. He was attached to his pole.

He was my first AIDS patient, a thirty-one-year-old homosexual who had been hospitalized many times. Drugs were being dripped into him via plastic tubing from high on the IV pole.

"It must be frustrating not being able to go anywhere," I suggested.

"No," he answered. "I calculated that twenty-two laps here equals one mile. I'm aiming to do three miles a day. Want some candy?"

"No, thank you."

He continued along his way, not to be interrupted.

Mr. Rainer wasn't the only patient to walk the hall. Three or four other patients would take themselves for a turn around the corridor, which formed a circular loop on the floor. They'd be spaced out at fairly even intervals, each a few doors down from the one ahead, as if in a continuous race.

As time went on, the more tests we performed on Mr. Rainer—blood cultures, radiologic studies, and eventually an open lung biopsy—the more depressed he became—and the more decorations he added to his IV pole. Soon there was a heart-shaped Mylar balloon that swayed a little behind him in the air as he sauntered along. Later, a white fluffy doll bobbed from the bottle hook.

Over the month he'd been there, he had accumulated a clutter of belongings, taping on his wall flowers, now withered, get-well cards, and paper plates he had colored with Crayola crayons. A friend of his had purchased the crayons in the hospital gift shop. The store didn't stock any other art supplies. The decorations resembled those in a third-grade elementary classroom. In retrospect, the makeshift and at times disorganized idiosyncrasy of his decorations may have been due to the AIDS virus causing a mild encephalopathy, an infection of the brain, which subtly alters one's visual-spatial judgment and perception. But he was a patient before researchers had learned how readily—yet subtly—AIDS can invade neurological tissue.

Mr. Rainer's face looked worn and hollowed from a loss of weight. AIDS patients, I was to learn, were often unkempt and unshaven, thin, with discolored cheeks and sunken eyes embedded in blackened rings. The virus made its victims grotesque, like sufferers of the bubonic plague.

Mr. Rainer, as an outpatient, had a private physician.

"I'm going to be in *The New England Journal of Medicine*,"

he told me gleefully one day. "Not me exactly, but my X rays. My private doctor just told me."

"Really?"

"Yeah, I always wanted to be in *The New England Journal of Medicine*." He paused and looked down. "Only I don't know if this is how I'd thought." Edward squeezed his eyebrows together but suddenly exclaimed, "Isn't that great?"

He didn't wait for a response, but quickly caught a nurse in the hall. "I'm going to be in *The New England Journal of Medicine*," I overheard him tell her.

When I entered his room the next day, he heaved himself forward in bed to sit up.

"Good morning, doctor. How are you doing today?" He attempted to transform my medical exam into a polite social call.

"Fine, thank you. But how are *you?*"

"I'm feeling better."

"How's your cough?"

"Mostly gone. My pneumonia must be almost all gone, huh?" He didn't say he had AIDS, only pneumonia—Pneumocystis. He didn't admit his infection was part of a disease spectrum. He hoped that after each hospitalization, his symptoms would remit. "I have a friend . . . actually someone I only heard about . . . who had Pneumocystis five years ago. He became macrobiotic, started to eat only certain foods, and has never been sick again. He must have had a complete remission. It happens."

Other AIDS patients acknowledged the disease more readily. "Don't shake my hand," one patient later warned me when I introduced myself to him. "They tell me I'm contaminated, you know."

"It's not transmitted by handshake," I said firmly, holding out my palm.

Mr. Rainer's parents came frequently to visit him. As he sat at the edge of his bed, they would sit on either side of him, like bookends, determined to be proud of their only son. Two male visitors also stopped in frequently, in vivid silk scarves and black leather boots. Their conversation was quickly suspended whenever I walked into the room.

Mr. Rainer's medical record showed that he had first developed diarrhea and night sweats. Many of his friends had already died of the disease. He knew what he had. But those initial symptoms had resolved a year ago. He took up yoga and even went to an ashram in Vermont. He took two months off from work to relax and adopted a macrobiotic diet, hoping that healthier eating habits would fortify his threatened immune system. He ate out only at the two restaurants in town that served whole grain rice, black beets, and beans. He felt in control of his diet, of what he gave his body to digest. He thought of emptying his bank account and traveling around the world, but decided to wait. Now, he was admitted with Pneumocystis carinii pneumonia, or PCP.

He was being treated with an antibiotic, Bactrim. If that didn't work, the next medicine tried would be pentamidine.

His pneumonia worsened.

"We're going to have to start you on the second drug," I told him.

He sadly shook his head. "Do I really need it?" We both knew he did.

He stopped doing laps. He stayed in his room, but kept up his spirits. "Do you think I'm getting better?" he'd ask each day.

"It's too early to tell."

One night when he spiked a fever, Walt, who was on call, entered his room to draw a blood culture. Walt carried three bottles of broth for culture medium with him, a bottle of Betadine that resembled a bottle of shampoo, and a pile of needles and alcohol swabs. He set all this equipment down on Edward's abdomen.

"You wouldn't believe it," Edward complained to me the next morning. "That other doctor came in and used me as a table!"

"How are you feeling now?"

"Oh, better. The fever must have been just a mild little thing."

Diane told me about one of the first AIDS patients they had had on the floor, about two years earlier, named Earl Grayson. He would brag to the staff about having had thousands of sexual encounters, as many as one hundred partners on a given weekend. The epidemic had sobered such talk. While Mr. Rainer admitted to being gay, there were patients who up until their last days continued to deny use of IV drugs, homosexual activity, ever receiving blood transfusions, or having had extramarital affairs. Their mode of transmission remained unknown, a secret carried to their graves.

When the first AIDS patients were admitted to the hospital, they were kept together on the fourth floor of a particular corridor that connected two other wings of the hospital. Residents and interns would often go from the fourth floor of one wing to the fourth floor of the other by going up one flight of stairs, across the connecting hallway on the fifth floor, and then down another stairwell back to four. They avoided having to walk through the AIDS ward, claiming that a patient had once had a bowel movement in the hallway. But fear of contagion can become emotional and irrational, even among the scientifically trained. Homophobia may play a role. "Rainer?" Walt once commented. "He's just another HIV player."

Edward had been admitted to a regular medical ward. Outside of his door, a cart was parked stocked with paper gowns,

hats, masks, shoes, and rubber gloves. Emmanuel and the
interns gloved up regularly. Diane was polite to him, but still
put on gloves before entering his room to avoid touching him.
The food service worker who dropped off his tray at mealtime
and picked it up afterward outfitted herself completely, even
with mask, hat, and paper shoe covers. The least educated
about the disease, she was the most frightened, and took the
most precautions.

The name of his disease has changed with medical understanding. Initially called Gay Related Immunodeficiency Disease, or GRID, the term was switched to Autoimmune
Deficiency Syndrome, or AIDS, when the disease process was
identified as a breakdown of the body's defenses. With the
discovery of a virus, patients were said to have "HTLV III,"
for Human T-Lymphocyte Virus, and later "HIV," for Human
Immuno-tropic Virus. Always an acronym. Always changing.

Diseases have often arisen from large-scale social changes.
Spanish explorers carried smallpox to the New World, dev-
astating Aztec and Incan populations, which lacked immunities
to it, and brought back syphilis to Europe, where, according
to some historians, it had never existed. The development of
better sanitation and indoor plumbing decreased early exposure
to the polio virus, thereby lowering levels of immunity in adults,
and instigating an epidemic. The sexual revolution created
opportunities for the spread of AIDS. The cost of social advance
can be disease.

Each year at the hospital, during Orientation Week, one or
two special lectures are given on topics of particular interest.
The year of my internship, the hospital lawyer presented a
special discussion on threats of legal action from patients. A
second lecture was on AIDS. These two topics seemed the
major ones of our times. The AIDS lecture briefed interns on
the latest research, urging a frightened audience that casual

contact with patients wasn't contaminating, and that rubber gloves, like condoms, could protect us. But we were provided with few answers as to how to cure Mr. Rainer or how to offer solace.

Mr. Rainer's pneumonia resolved. "How's he doing?" Emmanuel asked one morning as we stood by his bedside on rounds.

"He's stable. Status quo."

Mr. Rainer spoke up. "I can't help it if I'm boring."

"I think we can send you home tomorrow," I told him. That was the only genuinely positive remark I had been able to make to him during his stay.

"I guess I'm just a guy with nine lives," he said with a laugh. I forced a polite smile. We both knew this was only a respite. He'd be back someday soon.

The Man in the Pan

O ne day at home, Joseph Draper fell on the floor of his kitchen. He forbade his wife, Mabel, to call the doctor. They were an elderly couple who had lived a quiet life at home for many years. Their two daughters had grown up and moved away, and he had retired from the shoe repair shop where he had worked for forty years. Mr. and Mrs. Draper had grown old together.

One year earlier, a little past his seventieth birthday, Mrs. Draper noticed that her husband had a cough that had lingered for several weeks. It would start deep in his chest in spasms and rise until it erupted in his throat. "I'm taking you to the doctor, Joe."

"I don't want to see a doctor."

"You must." He still refused. She was small and frail. Though she was tough, she couldn't budge him. Finally she consulted the minister of her church, who encouraged her to persevere and suggested a ruse: she made an appointment for her husband and told him, "Joe, I'm going to see the doctor for myself. I want you to keep me company."

"What brings you here today?" Dr. Linden asked when they arrived.

"My wife," Mr. Draper replied.

"Let the doctor give *you* a checkup too," Mrs. Draper suggested. "Maybe he can help the cough."

Dr. Linden performed a routine physical exam and found some swollen lymph nodes. He ordered blood tests, and they revealed an abnormal number of white cells, and an elevated quantity of lactate dehydrogenase, an enzyme. Lymphoma was suspected, a cancer involving the lymph glands and white blood cells, which defend the body against disease. Mr. Draper was admitted to the hospital.

He had had a small heart attack years earlier and was a heavy smoker, but he now had a terminal illness. In his mind, though, his problem was only the cough, the only thing that he thought important. Not to Dr. Linden, who treated him with chemotherapy in the hospital and planned to continue it after discharge.

On the ward, Mr. Draper was poked and fingered, drugged, awoken and weighed. His wife wanted him to receive the best treatment, though he was indifferent. When he finally went home, he vowed never to return to the hospital. He refused appointments and never responded to the letters Dr. Linden's secretary mailed him. He was "lost to follow-up."

Untreated, his lymphoma burgeoned beyond control over the ensuing year until he collapsed on the floor of his kitchen. Unable to control his bodily functions, he lay paralyzed in feces and urine.

His wife phoned the police. When an ambulance arrived, the two medics wedged a stretcher underneath him and whizzed him back to the hospital. "Lord help me," he groaned as he arrived back on the ward.

Assigned as his intern, I introduced myself, but he didn't want to speak to me. He pinned his arms across his chest to both protect his body and prevent his blood pressure from being taken. He was on strike.

The blood-drawing team gave up trying to coerce him. It fell on me to coax him to let us sample his blood.

"Leave me alone. I don't want anything from you," he said.

"Mr. Draper, I need to draw some blood."

"I don't need it drawn." Emmanuel had acknowledged that my patient's disease might be too advanced to be helped by chemotherapy, but we were going to try to give him at least a few more weeks of life.

"We want to help you with your illness and your cough," I told Mr. Draper. Mabel was present and spoke up. "Come on, Joe. Do it for me."

"Okay," he said and sighed.

He also had shortness of breath, which I had to evaluate and consider treating. I telephoned a lab to schedule pulmonary function tests.

"You want PFTs?" the secretary repeated.

"Please."

"Patient's name?"

"Draper."

"He doesn't have any infectious diseases, does he? Anything like AIDS?"

"No, ma'am," I answered, surprised.

"Okay. We'll do him this afternoon at three. Send him over and don't forget his chart."

When Draper arrived, he refused to breathe into the machine. But finally he was persuaded, and puffed out his cheeks, straining into tubes that measured the strength and volume of his lungs.

The next day I stopped at his bed just after his dinner tray had been delivered. He was staring at the food, annoyed.

"What's wrong, Mr. Draper?" I asked.

"I asked for chicken," he complained. "I don't like meatloaf."

"I'll see what I can do," I said affably, and caught up with the tray cart down the hallway, where I managed to swap his dish for the choice he wanted.

This small favor led him to view me as a friend. If a nurse handed him any change in medications, he'd refuse. "I want to talk to my doctor first." He sensed that I was on his side and liked me even though he didn't understand the point of my tests—despite my explanations. Each morning he'd accost me with, "When are you going to let me leave, doc?" My resident and I were cautious, even though his cough had quieted down.

Joe would wander into the hallway when he wanted something. His thick black glasses weighed heavily on his sagging skin, and his hospital nightgown would be unsnapped in back and hang open. I would catch up to him and fasten the sides back together.

Late one night, his cough returned, along with shortness of breath. I lifted him onto a stretcher and trundled him down to the Radiology Department for an X-ray. By now the hospital had become a familiar environment to me. I knew where labs were located, enabling me to bring specimens there myself to save time, and which elevators were faster or slower.

The amount of oxygen and carbon dioxide in his blood also needed to be measured, by drawing a "blood gas," blood extracted from an artery. I poked a needle through the skin covering his radial artery on the undersurface of his wrist. I hurried, but no blood flowed. I struggled with the needle. He gritted his teeth. Most blood is drawn from veins, which bulge on the surface of the skin. An "arterial stick," as it's called, is more difficult and painful.

"Come on. Come on, doc. You can do it," he rooted. My brow sweated. He was praying to himself, his lips twitching, urging me on. Finally, our eyes widened as a track of blood crept up the clear plastic tubing toward my tube. Discovering oil couldn't be a greater relief. The two of us grinned at each other; it was the only time he ever smiled in the hospital.

"I think Joe should see a priest," his wife told me one day.

I relayed this to the ward clerk, who volunteered to call the hospital chaplain's office. She dialed a number. "Hello, this is Watkins-9," she said. "I'd like to arrange to have a prayer said for the patient in Room Nine-fifteen."

A minister in a black uniform arrived later that day, carrying a worn leather box and a computer printout of patients, listing their room numbers and religions. The box resembled an old shaving kit, but was filled with religious paraphernalia. Strings of yellow and pink rosary beads dangled over the edge.

Mr. Draper was angry at the intrusion.

"I want to go," he told me the next morning.

"Perhaps sometime soon if things start to go well, we can send you home."

"I want to go to die."

"But Mr. Draper, don't you want to live? We on the staff are going to help you stay alive longer." He shook his head.

I stopped Mrs. Draper and their two daughters in the hallway. "I'd like to sit down and talk to you for a few minutes, if you don't mind."

"Certainly, doctor."

I shepherded the family into a social worker's small office —a large closet, windowless but with plaid curtains strung on the wall, drawn closed to suggest the presence of a window. "As you know, Mrs. Draper, your husband has a life-threatening illness and might not have long to live. He may get more ill, and there are choices which we will have to make, perhaps on the spot, which we'd like to think about and prepare for ahead of time."

She nodded, quickly understanding what I was talking about.

Families usually do. "Specifically," I continued, "we like to talk to patients' families about how they feel about our taking heroic measures, if necessary to help him, such as special cardiac monitors."

"I know," she said. "I've seen it on TV." Television had also taught me the tone of the speech I was delivering. "Joseph's lived a good life," she said, sighing, "but he doesn't want to go on anymore, and I can't blame him. I don't want anything special done for him. You've all been helping him enough since he's become ill."

I wrote the order and Dr. Linden cosigned it.

"Mr. Draper is DNR. Thank God!" Diane exclaimed when the order had been written. "He's dying actively!"

To her, there seemed to be different ways of dying—actively and passively—even among chronic patients. One never heard the phrase "terminal cancer" mentioned in the hospital. Here, the issue was not whether a patient was terminal or not—we tried to treat all cancers. The question was only one of time, how much longer we would succeed in keeping a person alive. If failure was imminent, we let the patient go home or we changed his status.

A few days after I'd discussed these issues with Mr. Draper's family, Mr. Draper left for good.

I called Dr. Linden up at home to report his death. It was 1:00 A.M.

"Just get the family to consent to a 'post,' " Dr. Linden told me over the phone.

I had never had to get permission for an autopsy—a postmortem—before. I hunted for the appropriate form. Rita, who was on duty that night, directed me toward a dusty shelf stacked with batches of various administrative papers in manila folders.

I found the necessary form and brought it to the family. The three women, Mrs. Draper and the two daughters, leaned to- gether in an alcove by the elevator. A bag containing Mr. Draper's belongings stood on the floor beside them.

"I just spoke to Dr. Linden," I said. They raised their eyes toward me. How could I now transmit my curt phone conver- sation with Linden, where all he had said was to get them to consent to a "post." I would have to make something up. "He sends his sympathies," I offered.

"Oh thank you, doctor," Mrs. Draper gushed forth.

"I know it's a difficult moment for you, but he requested that I ask you if you would consent to an autopsy. We like to perform them on all patients. It tells us whether we missed anything which may help in the care of future patients."

"Will it hurt the way he looks?" she asked softly, gesturing to her face by moving her hand up and down in the air in front of it.

"No, it won't," I answered, although I had never actually seen a body after an autopsy was performed.

The women wanted to confer among themselves, and I left them alone.

In a few moments Mrs. Draper called me back.

"All right," she murmured. "You have our permission for the thing you're talking about."

"I need you to sign a form." I took out the consent statement. It was divided into three parts. The top read, "Autopsy." The second portion was headed "Donation of Eyes." The last part was for "Donation of Skin for Other Patients and for Research." She signed her name to the top section. "Would you like also to consider . . ." I pointed silently to the other two categories.

"No, that's enough," she said.

Two days later, the autopsy results were presented at Wednes- day morning pathology rounds. At these weekly meetings, the results of recent postmortem examinations are regularly shown and discussed.

I sat with Emmanuel, Walt, and Joan in the bleacher-like seats that ran along the back wall. In the front of the room there was a sunken pit in which a stainless steel pathology display table stood. On the floor beneath the table were drains; the table was hosed down after each use. In the background, a leaky faucet dripped into a sink, each plop echoing.

The pathologist, Dr. Spain, rolled out a cart stacked with what looked like cookie sheets. He pulled them out one by one and displayed them on the table. Each held a different organ. One tray exhibited the kidneys, another held slices of the liver neatly cut and laid out. "Here come the appetizers," Walt joked.

The conference is nicknamed "The Man in the Pan."

A cold air chilled my shoulders. My mind distanced these piles of flesh from the man who had been my patient, his brown eyes, and the smile I had once seen.

"Here is the heart," Dr. Spain announced in a deep and clear voice as he held up an irregular-shaped organ with cut flaps. "This is the aorta," he continued, poking a cold steel probe through various valves and holes till its shiny tip emerged at a distant port. I imagined the blood gushing along this now dry course, following the path of the silver tip. In our living chests the channels are wet. We all survive because of the push of blood each second following the trace of that metal finger.

The man I knew to be Mr. Draper and "the man in the pan" were materially the same, yet different—entities related by mere fact. I looked down at the table of trays. Now he was a pile of organs on bakery sheets.

I gazed from a distance at the heart. Once, Mr. Draper had offered me chocolates from a Whitman Sampler, a gift from his wife. His heart now flapped in a rubber glove, its mechanics demonstrated with tweezers. I saw a scorched part of the cardiac muscle, which had spasmed and died when a vessel clotted a few years earlier in a heart attack he had suffered. The tweezers scratched and tugged at the damaged wall of the heart, which had struggled too much.

"Here are the lungs." The pathologist pointed to a tray of thin, spongy, light brown slabs arrayed in decreasing size from the center to the edge of the cookie sheet. "We can see evidence of long-standing emphysema." Mr. Draper had been a heavy smoker. "We can feel how light and airy his lungs are," the pathologist said gaily. He demonstrated by raising one of the slices up and down in his hand, protected by a flesh-colored glove. These were the lungs that had coughed, bringing the patient to the hospital in the first place.

"These are diseased lymph nodes." He pointed to conglomerations of pale rubbery knots matted together, some blackened and hollow. Cancer is one of the diseases that look like a disease would be expected to look—disorganized, cruelly rotting away sleek and pearly organs. In lymphomas, the marks of destruction are subtler than in certain other kinds of cancer. "You can appreciate how close the tumor had come to wrapping itself around the great veins," Dr. Spain commented.

He dimmed the lights. Slides of microscopic cross sections of tumors were flashed on a screen. "These are boring, bland-looking cells," Dr. Spain commented. Each of the cells loomed before us on the overhead screen, thousands of times its actual size.

Dr. Spain displayed my patient's metastases sown like scattered seeds, purple and red-speckled, in other organs. "Note the bean-shaped nuclei of these other cells." Pathology uses many food names in its descriptions. Many diseased organs are reminiscent of types of food: both were once alive and follow organic patterns of growth. Cells split, fuse, swell, branch, reproduce, and become ill. Pathologists describe "nutmeg tumors" of the liver, "millet seed cavities" in tuberculosis, "cheesy necrosis," "cherry angiomata," "blueberry muffin lesions," and "Swiss cheese endometrium."

Later that day in the nursing station, a notice appeared thumb-tacked on a corkboard. It was a public invitation to attend a memorial service for Mr. Draper. The announcement cited him as "a generous and much loved member of our community." On the cover was a photograph of him which looked as if it had been taken several years ago, though it might have been only months before his death. He appeared healthier than I had ever seen him, wearing a jacket and tie and the same thick black glasses he'd worn in the hospital. I had difficulty imagining him in any other surroundings. For me, he had existed only on the ward.

A few weeks later, I received a carbon copy of the final autopsy report in my mailbox at the hospital, typed on thin crinkly tissue paper with a sharp blue margin. I felt disconnected from it as I held it between my hands, but in some physical sense it was him.

I still have the report.

Reverse Isolation

Albert Vier was a thirty-three-year-old fireman whom I met briefly one morning on rounds; later that day, when he spiked a fever, I went to reintroduce myself.

He was lying down, his torso raised, supported by his elbow, his light brown hair tousled. He waved me in and saluted me. "Yeah, right. Sure, we met. Hi, Bob," he called, spying my first name on my identification badge.

"How are you doing?"

"Okay. How are you doing?" It felt like the local bar.

"What's the score?" he asked.

"Huh?"

"Are you watching the game?"

"No, who's playing?"

"Chicago and Boston."

"Who are you rooting for?"

"Chicago's my team. We have to win this one big," he told me. Over his bed, he had hung up a pair of boxing gloves. He also had brought a TV from home, larger than the one provided

77

by the hospital, although it was turned off, and an exercise bicycle that he was too weak to use.

As I examined him and drew a blood culture, he told me that he'd played football in high school, and since he was a boy, had wanted to be a fireman stationed in the neighborhood where he had always lived.

He had leukemia and was receiving chemotherapy, which had destroyed his blood cells. The drug had put him quickly into remission, cutting down on the extraordinary number of cells exploding in his marrow, although it was killing good cells along with bad ones. A sample of his bone marrow had been removed and frozen for storage. His marrow was then blasted further with chemo to wipe it out altogether. Now, we were waiting for it to grow back. By the time he was assigned to me, he was "nadir," meaning that he had almost no cells left in his blood supply: few platelets, scant white blood cells, and an anemic level of red ones.

"What are my numbers today?"

"Your white count is zero point one." Normal is eight to twelve. He had close to nothing.

"It might start back up soon, doc, right?"

"Right, Mr. Vier."

The next day it was 0.2. He felt proud. But over the subsequent weeks, it didn't rise much higher. I gave him back his own marrow, to try to reseed his now vacant trabeculae, the intersecting pockets and tunnels in his bones' core. I waited for a few weeks, but the sowing failed to germinate. Meanwhile, he was anemic, having few platelets and lacking white cells to defend against disease. I transfused him with red cells and platelets almost daily. The latter are fragments formed when megakaryocytes, a family of bulging, monstrous blood cells, explode. Platelets patch up injured tissues, mending wounded walls of veins and arteries, and fight localized infections, summoning up more powerful white cells. White cells can't be transfused. They are finicky sentinels, identifying and loyally attacking the body's foes. They judge whether molecules they bump into are familiar or unknown, the product of self or stranger. They are xenophobic, ridding the bloodstream of foreign bodies. White cells from one person, if put into someone else genetically unrelated, will respond to the new body as an enemy and attack it. Everyone makes and needs his own white cells. Mr. Vier had none. Unless he started producing more of his own, he was in trouble.

Defenseless against invasion, he developed a persistent fever, a sign of possible infection. I added another antibiotic. The fever continued, and a second and then a third antibiotic were employed. Eventually amphotericin, an antifungal agent, was begun. This drug of last resort was potent but destructive, inflicting many side effects. It made patients feel, as one said, "sick as shit," inducing bouts of nausea and vomiting lasting for hours. The drug slashed even further the numbers of Mr. Vier's white blood cells and platelets, decimating these troops. The body was weakened before becoming stronger. In an effort to fight disease, it was first rendered defenseless.

Mr. Vier's vulnerable body grew frail. The tiniest bedsore or scratch or popped pimple festered into a purple-ringed hole on his surface. To touch his own skin was painful and dangerous.

He was kept in Reverse Isolation. Precautions were taken to prevent others from inadvertently infecting him. Nothing that wasn't sterile was allowed to touch him.

His wife came to visit several times a week. Pretty and provocatively dressed, she looked as if she would have liked to be alone with him. But physical contact between them wasn't possible. His food, too, had to be sterile and he was on an Isolation Diet. His meals were shipped to the floor specially prepared and sealed in plastic wrap on disposable paper trays with white plastic implements. Even cookies came sterilely wrapped with "904," his room number, penned on the plastic wrap with Magic Marker.

Every day, Emmanuel and I would put on paper gowns and enter his room. Above his bed, a stethoscope was specially kept dangling on a hook, staying germ free. But it was often misplaced and I had to use my own.

In that case, I had to protect him from the bulb of my stethoscope, which had touched other patients' skin, I inserted the small drum at the end of the scope into my palm inside my sterile glove. With this receiver cupped in my hand I listened to the noises made by his heart and lungs. His heart beat through the plastic skin of both the glove and the drum. My whole hand explored his back and chest. I had ears in my fingers. To listen better, I didn't bend or turn my head, I moved my whole arm.

After a few long weeks in isolation, he grew more depressed. "Can't I go for a walk around the ward?" he asked one day. I shook my head. "The nursing station and back? Please?" he whispered softly. I wanted to take him beyond the threshold of his door, but couldn't.

"I'm sorry, Mr. Vier," I said through the paper mask covering my face. The paper suspended over my mouth muffled my voice. I inhaled the acerbic smell of antiseptic. "Thank you, though." I sighed. He hadn't done me a favor except allowing me to examine him but I felt the need for some warmth between his imprisoned machismo and my white coat, acknowledging at least the illusion of one of us benefiting the other.

"Wait . . . " he called as I neared the door. "What time is it?"

"What time would you guess?" I responded, testing how oriented he was.

"I have no idea. Six o'clock?"

"Morning or evening?"

"I don't know. Morning, maybe?"

"It's nine in the morning," I had to say, sad to have had to quiz him to assess his confusion. "Do you know what day it is?" I asked.

Embarrassed, he didn't, and I told him.

Posted on the wall was a large calendar on which he or his wife crossed off each day.

The next morning, the date had been circled in thick red ink.

"What day is it?" I inquired again.

"It's September . . ." He strained to peek at the calendar.

"No cheating now, Mr. Vier."

"September something." He still didn't know.

He remained on the ward because of his marrow's sluggish rebound. But he got depressed again. "Mr. V.'s looking down," his nurse, Diane, said one day. "Maybe you can call a psych consult." The nurses asked house officers for a psychiatry consultation on most oncology patients at one point or another. The request often signaled that the nurses themselves were demoralized and distraught with the patient. Most interns didn't bother to consult a psychiatrist unless the problem was severe, though it was usually helpful when the intern did call, legitimizing the staff's frustration and benefiting the patient.

"I'm giving him a heavy dose of flirt therapy," Diane confessed to me. "Two weeks ago he was saying he wanted to die. It's worked. He's perked up and says he won't give up hope." She smiled.

But over subsequent weeks, his white count didn't advance.

When my rotation on the ward came to a close, I went to say goodbye to him.

"Doctor, I'll be all right, don't you think?" He looked searchingly in my eyes.

"I hope so."

"Can't I leave the room with you just for a moment?"

"I'm afraid not."

"What could possibly happen?" I feared invisible germs that might be hovering outside his sterile room. "Why am I here? Please . . ."

"No. I'm sorry."

That was the last conversation I ever had with him. Allowing him to leave his cell, even for seconds, would have meant more to him than the drugs and blood transfusions that I had labored to provide.

I don't know what happened to Mr. Vier after I left Watkins-9. I don't know if he ever made it to the hall.

Requests

"I have another hit coming up from the ER," Walt told the nurse, Rita. "Elnora Fields. A multisystem failure who's got neurological problems."

"Is she a walkie-talkie?"

"She's a talkie, but not a walkie. She doesn't move much."

"Which room is she going into?"

"How about across from that dirtball patient, Craw? He's still pretty gorked out,"—meaning comatose—"isn't he?"

"He's beginning to wake up."

"Let's stick her there anyway." Mr. Thomas Craw was an alcoholic and an IV drug abuser with liver disease and diabetes who had overdosed. The police had found him in the gutter. Several times he had been warned to obtain treatment for his drug addiction. Once, he had enrolled in a detoxification and rehabilitation program that had kept him "clean" for six months. But he had returned to his drugs. "Heroin is his drug of choice," Walt had once announced as if speaking about his brand of breakfast cereal or beer.

In the morning, Walt described Mrs. Fields on rounds. "She's an obese seventy-year-old black female who presents with multisystem failure—cardiovascular disease, diabetes, strokes, and end-stage renal disease." Her kidneys were giving up. "Every six months she comes in to be tuned up," meaning her medications were fiddled with in response to her episodes of crisis. "It's all catching up with her lately. She goes to renal dialysis to get spun in the washing machine there three times a week." He listed her multiple medications, including aspirin to "grease her platelets"—that is, to impede them from clotting and precipitating another stroke. "She is," he added on the side, "a 'Lord Have Mercy-er.' "

"What's that?" I inquired.

"She always says 'Lordhavemercy, Lordhavemercy.' " He spoke each phrase as a one-word sigh.

Indeed, muffled from behind her face mask, those were the words we heard when we crowded around her bed. She lay stranded on her mattress.

There, in the ICU, Mr. Craw and she developed a dialogue of sorts, each hardly cognizant of anything around them.

"Lordhavemercy," she cried.

Mr. Craw, barely awake to this world, his eyes still half closed, rolled his head back and forth.

"Doctor!" he groaned. "Hey you, nurse. Get over here!" he'd stammer out as, from the corner of his eye, he thought he saw something moving.

"Lord, Lord, Lord," Mrs. Fields would plead.

"Fuck the Lord."

"Lordhavemercy!"

"Fuck mercy! Fuck doctors! I want to get out of here. NURSE!" He shook the IV stand next to him. "Are you listening to me?" he yelled at the pole, rattling it more after each failure to respond. "Are you listening to me?" He raised his voice each time, incensed.

No one responded except Mrs. Fields. Over the next few nights and days, they'd periodically awaken each other.

"Lordhavemercy," she'd chant. Their conversation would start again. Every few hours, they'd exchange their exclamations, the only ones to acknowledge each other's requests. No nurse or doctor answered them when they each feebly chanted for help.

A few days later, a friend of Mr. Craw's showed up, in his mid-thirties, unshaven with shaggy black hair. His leather jacket was encrusted with patches from Hell's Angels, and his black boots were caked with mud. At the cuff of his right arm protruded not a hand but a prosthetic device, metal robotic prongs clutching a motorcycle helmet. He had continued to cycle after losing his arm. In his other hand, he lugged a large radio which he lent to the patient. When Mr. Craw's stupor began to clear, he wailed to songs. Unable to carry a tune, he moaned "Jumping Jack Flash" and "I Can't Get No Satisfaction." It was time that he moved out of the ICU to a regular room. But he decided not to wait for his health to be fine-tuned.

One morning Walt told me, "Craw's A.M.A.," meaning he had signed out Against Medical Advice. He'd return someday if the police bumped into him in time.

Mrs. Fields was also transferred out of the unit onto the ward once she was stabilized. Her condition was still precarious. I balanced her glucose and titrated several medicines for her heart, lungs, and kidneys. But I was battling against natural forces. In addition, she still couldn't walk. As a professor told me, by the time a patient's denial breaks down and he or she comes to the hospital, he has exhausted his reserves—psychological as well as physical. To be sick means to have used up one's resources.

This professor had told me that the Social Work Department had once done a follow-up study of what former patients thought years later of the treatment they had received in the hospital, how they looked back on it, what they remembered most. The ones who could walk all gloated, "See, they said I wouldn't be able to walk, and I can." The ones who couldn't grumbled, "They said I'd be able to walk, and I can't." In fact, the professor told me, neither had been said except that outcomes weren't predicted well.

Emmanuel told me to have the social worker "get on the case" of Mrs. Fields. Judy Aaron was the social worker assigned to the floor, a tall woman with braided hair and earrings of chunky pieces of plastic and a thick loose-leaf notebook in which she wrote everything down.

I walked up to her in the nursing station. "On Mrs. Fields, the resident asked if we could get social services involved in planning her discharge."

"Is this 'Let's involve them today,' meaning they should have started yesterday?"

"No," I answered ignoring the sharp barb. "Whenever you get a chance." Some interns and residents perceived the ward social worker as having a much smaller volume of work than they, despite her frequent complaints of being "dumped on." But she seemed to me to work hard, mending family animosities and financial problems.

"How are you doing?" I asked Mrs. Fields the next day.

"Lordhavemercy."

"Any problems?"

"My leg."

"Which leg?"

"The left one."

"What's the matter?"

"It's in pain."

In her fat calf, I palpitated and rolled between my fingertips a ropelike cord, a vein clogged from blood slogging in its amble back to her heart, slowed by her leg unmoving between the

sheets. If blood coagulates in a calf, it may plug up an arteriole
in the lung too, as a potentially fatal pulmonary embolus.
Another drug, Coumadin, was started to thin her blood. This
chemical, the trademark version of sodium warfarin, is commonly used as rat poison, making rodents bleed to death.

"Does anyone live with you?" I asked a few days later.

"Nobody but me." No one even visited her in the hospital.
Her husband had died ten years before.

"Do you have any children?" I asked, thinking of possible
caretakers outside of the hospital.

"A daughter."

"Is she nearby?"

"She's living across town; but she doesn't come around to
see me much."

I wondered where she would go when she left here. Since
she was barely able to get out of bed, I thought I might have
to send her to an "an adult home," as nursing homes were
called. The deep vein thrombosis in her leg portended con-
finement in bed. She wasn't getting any better. "It's only a
matter of time," Emmanuel told me. Because of her poor prognosis, she was made DNR.

A week later, when I was on call, Rita paged me. "You
need to pronounce Mrs. Fields."

The alcove of the pale yellow chamber glowed in fluorescent
light. On her night stand, a pasty Jesus Christ looked up and
out from a wooden frame. Splayed out from his head were white
flanges tipped with red, representing a flaming halo and resembling the tentacles of a sea creature. A pastel blue sky lay
flat and oppressively behind him. Religious pictures positioned
by a patient's bedside can be an ominous sign, often denoting
that the patient is faring badly.

Mrs. Fields's enormous body lay still as if asleep. The room
was nearly dark. There was no sound of her loud, wet, sonorous

breathing, or her plaintive cry. From the doorway of the silent room, I knew what had happened. As officially required, I would examine her anyway, not wanting to miss anything as significant as life.

Though I had unconsciously dismissed her cry as an empty phrase, its meaning now became clear. From her mouth, it was neither idle nor profane. It was prayer.

Back in the nursing station, I walked past Emmanuel. "Did you pronounce her?" he asked.

"Yes." I paused, hesitant to tell him the thoughts I had had in her room. Would he think me too sentimental, emotional, or religious? No physician wanted another to suspect him of being anything less than logical. But I had experienced a feeling in her room that had captured her state, embodying some inherent truth. "The one thought I had," I confessed, "was that the Lord had mercy on her."

Emmanuel looked at me, smiled, and said, "He did."

A Year-long Night

"Are you the doctor in charge?" a young woman in jeans asked me in the hallway one evening.

"I'm the doctor on call . . . yes." Every third night, this was my role. I was Beeper 81.

"Oh, thank God," she exclaimed. Her hair was too shiny and her skin too clear for her to be a patient. "Can you come see my mother?"

"Who's that?"

"Georgine McDonald."

I had admitted her mother to the hospital a few days earlier.

"I'm Dr. Klitzman."

"Sue McDonald."

"What's the matter?"

"She's not looking too well." Mrs. McDonald had breast cancer disseminated to bone and brain. Her attending physician had made her DNR when he admitted her to the ward.

"Okay. But I won't be able to stop by for a few minutes.

There's an emergency I have to take care of first." I started to step away.

"I just want someone to tell me how much longer she has to live," Miss McDonald continued. "One month or six months. Partly so my sister and I can start making . . . plans . . . you know." I was surprised not by her wanting to know but by the fact that she was bringing this up now, slipping it in as if it were an emergency or a question that would yield a short and easy answer.

"Let's talk about that when I come back up." My feet carried me away.

Family members seek predictions, but I'd been instructed not to divine the future. The course of most diseases is too erratic. Furthermore, families visit patients in the evening after work, after most of the medical staff has gone home for the day. When I'm on call, I end up consoling and updating families of certain patients I barely know, since their care is really the responsibility of the other two interns.

When I entered Mrs. McDonald's room she was coughing up globs and gushes of blood, which Sue blotted with a wrinkled Kleenex.

"Do you know where you are?" I asked her mother. I had posed this question each day. She usually stared at me silently and blinked, unable to answer. I repeated the query now, expecting no response.

But she suddenly turned to her daughter, who hadn't been present at the previous inquiries. Mrs. McDonald's lips parted. "There he goes again," she stammered. I was thunderstruck. She had been mute for weeks.

"Where are you?" I repeated. She smacked her lips.

This question was standard for assessing orientation and detecting delirium. I once asked it of a patient awakening from coma. She arched herself up on her elbows, scanned the room, and whispered with perplexed embarrassment, "Heaven?"

"What's your *name?*" I asked Mrs. McDonald. She puckered her lips, making a sucking noise, but she didn't respond. Her daughter held her mother's shoulders, urging her on. I shook my head. "She doesn't look good, but she seems stable."

"I just wanted someone to see her, doctor. She's here all alone, you know," Sue said, and followed me into the hallway. "How long does she have to live?"

"It's hard to say. Each patient is different. We're not good at predicting." I never felt comfortable being the one to set these prognoses, these purchases of time. Whatever period I threw out would be forever chiseled in her daughter's mind.

Over the ensuing weeks, I greeted Sue McDonald whenever I was on call. One evening, Rita paged me. "McDonald's daughter wants to see you again."

It was a busy night. "Tell her that I'll try to come by later." I was drawing blood from another patient. Just then, the page operator's voice echoed throughout the emptied hallways of the hospital—*The Department of Medicine Nutrition Conference is now beginning in the D-Seven Meeting Room.* It was 9:00 P.M. I thought of Miss McDonald waiting, but rationalized venturing downstairs briefly. I would be able to be more attentive to her needs afterwards.

"Nutrition Conference" is the code phrase for supper, perhaps my only break of the night. When I arrived downstairs, a cluster of interns huddled around a table piled with white cardboard cartons of Chinese food, gulping down forkfuls. We ate out of blue, kidney-shaped plastic tubs known as "Gomer Bowls," pulled off the ward's utility cart and normally used to collect the secretions of severely ill patients. The containers came individually wrapped in plastic, sterilized and costing the hospital much more than paper plates, which weren't provided.

We consumed the food standing up, aware that we could be called away at any second by our beepers clasped to our hips.

The food itself was often supplied by a drug company representative, pleased to be able to make our night more comfortable at the behest of his firm. Drug representatives filtered through the hallways of the hospital, and various interns and residents befriended them. When I strode down the hall a man in a gray business suit would occasionally catch my eye and put down his briefcase with a metal click. "You look like a house officer," he'd greet me, extending his hand. I'd know who he was immediately. Walt seemed particularly adept at cultivating these relationships. The salesmen would hail him as if they had been old friends. Walt was continually supplied with new ballpoint pens bearing the name of an expensive antibiotic, Valium paperweights, Keflex pads of paper, Kefzol penlights and Cardizem mugs.

"How's it on Morgan-Ten?" I asked another intern, Erica Chin. She was standing beside me as we waited to press in toward the food table.

"It's bad, real bad," she answered.

"Oh?"

"I'm being killed. I just had a patient code on me."

"What happened?"

"He's at the funeral parlor now." She glanced over toward the Chinese food, still three people away. Most codes fail, though one revival can compensate for the labor of countless losses. To Erica, coding was synonymous with death.

"What was the story?"

"He was a real scumbag who crashed. He went into respiratory arrest. I called a code but it didn't do anything."

"Have things quieted down since then?"

"Are you kidding?" She made me feel foolish for even asking. "I've already had three admissions. I wish it were a full house. There are still eight open beds. Also, my resident is a real pump." Residents stationed in the Emergency Room who decided whether patients would be admitted or not fell into three categories: "walls" managed to keep patients out of the hospital, arranging for many to be treated as outpatients; "sieves" permitted patients to come into the hospital easily; "pumps" pushed people in who didn't have to be admitted. "I just hope nothing else comes into the ER," she said. She suddenly shoved through the crowd, shouldering her way toward the table.

I watched Erica disappear into the throng of interns massed around the food as I waited my turn. Each night on call I hoped for a quiet evening, and reminded myself that no matter how busy the night, it would end within twenty-four hours. In retrospect, I realize that I learned the most at night, deciding how to tackle new crises.

My beeper abruptly emitted a series of high-pitched squeals. In the course of an on-call night, my beeper might erupt twenty or thirty times. I sought out the nearest phone, not yet having reached the table, and dialed the ward. Mathilda answered.

"It's Bob," Mathilda squawked through the nursing station. "Anyone page him?"

Rita, the night nurse, had summoned me. "Mrs. Rodriquez is having chest pain," she stated flatly. This constituted a medical emergency. I rushed back upstairs, hoping leftovers might be available later.

Mrs. Rodriquez's bed was isolated at the far end of the hallway.

"Dr. Klitzman . . . ?" Miss McDonald tried to engage me in the hallway.

"I'll have to talk to you later, okay?" I continued on.

The wind whistled past Mrs. Rodriquez's window as I staggered in. Outside, the lights of the city twinkled. Above her head shone a single overhead lamp.

"How are you doing?"

"I'm having chest pain," her frail lips muttered. Her face was pale.

"Where on your chest?" She pointed. "Does it radiate anywhere?"

She shook her head.

"Shoulders? Neck? Arms?"

"No."

"Any nausea? Shortness of breath?"

I asked these routine questions automatically. She was sixty-seven years old and had had a myocardial infarction, a heart attack, six years earlier. She had been admitted several times since, most recently a few days ago, complaining of chest pain again. Her tests on these subsequent admissions were negative, showing that her discomfort wasn't caused by her heart. Her pain now was again probably indigestion or her imagination but I'd have to check.

The first time I had to manage a patient with chest pain, Emmanuel had accompanied me to the bedside and demonstrated how to examine the patient: how to pose questions, record and decipher a portable EKG, administer sublingual nitroglycerin, and remeasure the patient's blood pressure. "See one, do one, teach one," he had announced, citing a commonly invoked principle of clinical education. "Next time you'll be doing all this by yourself." The neophyte is quickly expected to be able to instruct others. Assistance is occasionally required and provided. But this often quoted motto establishes a tone and standard that ignores a beginner's anxiety, doubt, or clumsiness.

I listened to Mrs. Rodriquez's heart thumping. A light swish followed every other pound—a faint heart murmur. My mind reviewed the endless list of tasks that awaited me, including speaking with Sue McDonald. I concentrated on the first heart sound and then the second. I glanced at her chart and noted that in Walt's admission note, beside the heading "cor," standing for coronary, the following string of coded letters was scrawled: "nl. s1, s2, no s3, s4, + II/VI se(m), no g, r." The symbols communicated that she had had a normal first heartbeat, a normal second one, and no extra third or fourth beat. She had a systolic ejection murmur that was rated with a score of two, on a scale from zero to six, with six representing a murmur that could be heard without a stethoscope. She had no cardiac gallops or rubs. Based on this coded description, her heart exam hadn't changed. I listened through her back. The wind howled in the caverns of her lungs. I went into the hallway to bring in an EKG machine, and graphed her heart's electrical rhythm. After I administered nitroglycerin, easing the root-beer-colored tablet under her tongue like a coin, her pain vanished. I sighed in relief. Still, the improvement could have been due to either the drug or a spontaneous resolution of the discomfort. I pierced one of her veins with a needle to the depth that let blood flow like juice into my glass tubes to measure a fresh set of enzymes.

Back at the nursing station, I wrote orders for the morning: a second set of enzymes and a second EKG.

As I headed off, Rita spotted me. "You have another admission coming up," she said. It was my third.

"Jesus," I mumbled to myself.

"It must be a full moon tonight," she commented wryly.

"They say it's always a full moon over Watkins-Nine," Mathilda commented without looking up. Disaster wasn't odd or even exceptional here, but lurked constantly. I could never imagine other interns performing the tasks that confronted me when I was on call. Each of my nights seemed a unique hell, the unfolding of unforeseen crises.

My beeper started squeaking spasmodically again, telling me to phone the Emergency Room. I dialed the number.

"Dr. Klitzman, returning a page."

"Toot, toooot," a voice answered.

"Is this the ER?"

"Yes, it's Emmanuel." He laughed. "There's a train wreck for you to admit down here. You might want to come down to eyeball her."

He told me about the case. "You seem to have a black cloud over you," he told me. Ordinarily scientific-minded, he was superstitious about the hardships of working in a hospital. "You have the worst luck," he told me. House staff—interns and residents—were incessantly comparing each other's "luck." When on call, I was at the mercy of unpredictable events. I could secure anywhere from eight hours of sleep to none, determined by how many problems happened to transpire during the night. I would lie quietly in the on-call room, reading, not knowing whether my beeper would startle me in the next minute or not until the next morning. What I told myself in order to feel more in control was that each event presented a potential opportunity to learn. But at 4:00 A.M. my motivation for education was at its nadir.

As I spoke with Emmanuel, I thought of bloods that remained to be drawn, lab values from earlier in the evening to check, orders to write, and drugs to administer. Mrs. McDonald was fast slipping from my mind. I resigned myself to having missed dinner. Before Walt and Joan had left for the day, they had each handed me an updated "sign-out sheet," listing all of their patients, a brief blurb about each one, and any tasks that would need to be done. Walt's sheet was sloppy and quick. "Hold down the fort, buddy," he said to me, slapping my back as he handed me the piece of paper. "Don't let them hurt you too bad."

I had a few minutes before the admission arrived on the floor. My first job was to give an injection to a patient through her IV tubing. I slurped up the fluid with a syringe in the medication station. Her room was next door. In filling the syringe, I accidentally misplaced the protective needle cap. I decided to carry the needle carefully across the hall without it. My hand screened it as I proceeded cautiously.

"You shouldn't be walking around with that needle unsheathed," Rita chided me. I was spotted.

"I know, I'm just bringing it to the room right here."

"You know, you know, but you don't do," she snapped. She bossed around patients, other nurses, and young doctors alike. She truckled to none and terrorized any who stood in her path. I continued on my way. My agenda beckoned.

I wondered about her choice to work only these dismal hours between 11:00 P.M. and 7:00 A.M., when everyone should be asleep. Another nurse, Jennifer, occasionally assumed a few of these night shifts in exchange for day shifts she wanted free. Nurses with seniority avoided the hours altogether. But for Rita, only the night mattered. The night shift was her life. During these hours, she was in control. She'd choose to notify me as to how patients were managing. If I voiced annoyance, she'd harass me for the remainder of her time of duty. She'd pester me with insignificant reminders and irrelevant facts, such as that someone's vital signs remained normal. "Watch out," Walt would remind me, "Rita's on tonight. She can hurt you."

Interns envied the nurses their ability to leave the hospital promptly at the end of an eight-hour shift, no matter what problems remained unresolved. Nurses knew when they'd return home. As a point of honor, most interns upheld the code of ethics that they would finish as much work as they could before departing at the end of the day and try to avoid abandoning incipient disasters. Interns who failed to do this were rebuked.

Nurses, for their part, envied doctors for their power and their mobility. Interns were still rising through their profession.

Some nurses had witnessed interns become attendings, and move on and eventually out of the hospital. Most registered nurses were stable or stuck in their jobs, with little chance of advancement. A few might become head nurses. In the beginning of the year, nurses knew more than interns about some aspects of the logistical management of patients—what forms needed to be completed, how to order tests. By now, four months into the year, these positions were reversed.

At 10:00 P.M., a band of three musicians sauntered through the ward like wandering minstrels. An aging woman with dyed blond hair played an accordion as she sang. A white cowboy hat was tied to her chin. An older, shorter man with sunken cheeks and a checked shirt strummed a banjo. A tall man with gray hair and a pot belly picked a guitar, wearing a brick red cowboy hat and a blue-sequined vest. They strolled down the hall, stopping in front of patients' rooms. They serenaded a senile alcoholic, who clapped his hands to their melody and bobbed his bald head back and forth, his bony shoulders swinging like a metronome out of sync.

By the time I had a free moment and headed into Mrs. McDonald's room, it was too late to see her daughter; visiting hours were over.

At 2:00 A.M., I completed my list of chores and "worked up" yet another admission. I consulted the sign-out sheets handed to me earlier by Walt and Joan, making sure everything had been done, and crawled off to the on-call room to find refuge. In the center of this tiny cubicle, which doubled as an examining room, was a table complete with stirrups for gynecological checkups. In the corner was crammed a fold-up cot, my bed, my island of rest. Above me, a glass cabinet displayed the remains of a collection of bottles and white plastic buckets of disposable instruments. One side of the cabinet was labeled "pelvic," the other side, "procto."

On the windowsill were piled long-forgotten medical charts of discharged patients. If and when these patients were ever readmitted, the Medical Records Department would report that the charts from the previous hospitalizations were "missing." Old tubes of blood were scattered about, many lacking identifying labels.

On the wall was a hand-lettered poster which read: "Seventy percent of patients get better on their own." Penciled in on the side was the addendum "Yeah and God saves the other thirty percent." Another intern had printed in large letters at the bottom, "Ten percent will die anyway." Throughout medical school, professors jokingly informed us of the "one-third rule." One third of patients get better, one third get worse, and one third stay the same, no matter what the disease or treatment.

Now, with my work complete, I lay down to sleep. I tossed in the narrow cot, wondering if anyone would die tonight, if my decisions had all been correct. The restless nights and dreams of other interns over the years lurked in the room. Merely knowing that I could be roused at any moment by a crisis hampered my rest. Internship had hardened me, enabling me to survive with little sleep, to overcome my body's instinctual resistance to being awoken and thrust into work. I became efficient enough at my job to eke out a few hours of sleep from most nights. But each night seemed endless, each a year long. Time would slow down. I often ceased to believe I'd see the light of day again.

Soon, though, I was asleep.

At 4:00 A.M. Rita paged me. "You have to pronounce the patient McDonald."

In an empty daze, my body mechanically stood up, slipped on my sneakers, and stumbled out of the dark room into the fluorescent-lit hall. I crept into Mrs. McDonald's room. Her death did not come as a surprise. On a ward with cancer patients, as many as three deaths might occur on a single evening. At her bedside leaned a framed photograph of her in a bright red dress and a bouffant hairdo.

I pronounced her.

Half an hour later, Rita paged me again. A demented patient named Bayer had squirmed free from her IV. Medication poured through the line. I bustled into her room to open a vein. I had never met her before but had heard about her case. She shook to escape my fingers as they probed her limbs for a vessel. She wiggled and thrashed to flee the posey into which she was strapped, a vest tied loosely to the side rails, used for patients who are agitated and might otherwise fall out of bed. Rita held her down. Mrs. Bayer bleated, but finally yielded and bent her arm so I could pierce a wobbly vessel. With the task done, I started to back away when I spotted a symmetrical bulge lying over her trachea. I palpated it with my fingertips. "Is that a mass on her neck?" I asked Rita.

"It's been there since she's been in," Rita answered bluntly. The patient's problem was long-standing, my presence fleeting. This was my one and only encounter with Mrs. Bayer. I didn't even know her first name.

"Do you know if there's any food around?" I asked Rita.

"You're just going to have to wait until the morning." It was 5:00 A.M. I stumbled into the kitchen on the ward anyway and opened the cold stainless steel doors of the walk-in refrigerator.

A cloud of cold, wet vapor enveloped me. Inside, carts were lined up supporting stacks of trays on rungs that enabled them to slide in and out easily, morguelike. I was prohibited from deserting the ward and was hungry and weary, and desperate to satisfy at least one of those basic needs. I felt frozen and numbed in the surgical scrub suit I wore when on call. The low V-neck of the loose shirt stuck to my chest. The baggy pants clung to me, weighed down by a heavy beeper.

I held open the cold latch and crouched down, peering one rung at a time into the trays of half-eaten meals left by the sick. I stared vacantly, my stomach empty, my eyes red and dry. Many of the meals were low-salt diets or bland renal diets of minuscule amounts of protein, allocated to patients who had had kidneys excised or transplanted. The meals would be tasteless, but they were food.

Suddenly, I noticed that one meal tray was intact. It probably hadn't been given to its claimant, and hadn't left the cart since being placed there twelve hours earlier in the main kitchen of the hospital. Here was virgin food, untouched by sick hands. I slid the tray halfway out and unfolded a small slip of paper positioned in front of the main dish.

Room 919, it read. *McDonald*.

I pulled the tray out all the way, and weighed it in my hands. It would have been her last supper. I looked down at the plastic cutlery, the covered main dish.

I shuffled into the on-call room and dropped the tray onto the examining table. This was going to be breakfast, I decided. It was better than nothing. I thought of Mrs. McDonald as I unwrapped the utensils, sealed in cellophane, picturing her hoary curls and her blue eyes' speechless gaze.

I had been reduced to a scavenging beast, an automaton. My intellect still functioned, though at a slightly slowed speed. I was emotionless and guiltless, barren and icy. Survival first.

I hadn't bothered to heat the food in the microwave in the kitchen. I stabbed the prongs of the fork into the main course.

It was the coldest meal I ever ate.

Radiology Suite

Every afternoon, my resident, the other interns, a troop of medical students, and I descended on the Radiology Department. We nabbed all the swivel chairs in the room and spun them over to the corner where our patients' films were stored and displayed.

Dr. Flint presided, a radiologist with thick gray-streaked hair and glasses. He wore a white button-down shirt every day, but unlike those who spent time on the ward with patients, he never donned a white coat.

He would stare at the films on his board like a magician, a seer of the invisible. The machine would grind as his foot pressed a pedal and churned the loop of films around and around. "There," he'd say as the picture we had requested to see rolled into view.

It was important to see the films directly, because Dr. Flint's readings of them were often cryptic. More than any other branch of medicine, radiology has been guilty of obscuring its findings through its language. Radiologists describe their observations vaguely, cautiously. "The possibility of a tumor may not perhaps be entirely excluded," he had written about one patient's study. The comment failed to tell me whether the patient had cancer or not.

An X-ray cuts through flesh to see the common denominator of bones. Everybody's skeleton is essentially identical. Fragile bones encase dark spaces which are vulnerable to disease. Lungs are blasted by dusty air filled with lint and bacteria. Viruses and spores get sucked into our mouths with every inspiration.

Reading X-rays is an art. Subtly different gray tones of intersecting ovals, oblongs, circles, and teardrops are created by overlapping body parts. These forms confound each other and meld into odd, dark shapes that can be mistaken for abnormalities. A small rounded blob might be a diseased lymph node or a tumor, which is then thought to exist because it was spotted, clearly circumscribed, on a photograph. Dr. Flint could tap the eraser tip of his pencil on its milky outline. His eye was caught by and followed various planes of hue. "These are suspicious shadows," he would say prophetically. "I think there's something there, though it might be a 'soft call,' " as opposed to a pronouncement more rooted in "hard" empirical data, the stuff of a truly "hard" science, believed to be more characteristic of the physical than the behavioral sciences. After looking at thousands of examples, Dr. Flint became trained to pick out the relevant from the background—to discriminate between real findings and artifacts of the study itself. "You find what you look for," Dr. Flint once confessed, "and you look for what you know."

Walt had his own adage about the field. "Whenever you see an arrow penned onto an X-ray," he confided once, referring to X-rays that had already been read and marked up by a radiologist, "there's a good chance there's an abnormality there."

After viewing a patient's serial films snapped over successive days, I begin to recognize him or her by his X-rays. From a row of chests, each with vaulting ribs splayed like fans, and spines gently notched like bamboo by the indentations of vertebrae, I had been able to pick out the chest of my first patient, Victoria Steiner. The pole of her spine was squat, the spread of ribs leaned to one side, that of her broken arm. Her clavicles tilted. I could recognize her ribs, and even the vacuous spaces of her lungs sprinkled with gray and white specks, and threads imprinted by her arterioles, and her faint lymphatic channels. One patient's identifying sign was the shadow of a gold necklace strung around her neck on each film as day to day her pneumonia improved, as gray clouds accumulated and then dissipated in the lower right corner. The gold jewelry left a white shadow. Another patient's tumor, between her third and fourth ribs on the left, changed from the size of a tennis ball to a squash ball to a cherry to a pea over ensuing weeks of chemotherapy.

Once, after Miss Steiner had died, I happened on an X-ray of her chest lying on a table in the back room of the ICU where she had spent a critical stretch of her last days. "Victoria Steiner" it read in the corner. Held up to the light, her congestive heart failure loomed larger than while she was on our ward. Fluid had collected in the costophrenic angles, the gutters on each side of the chest where the diaphragm muscle supporting the base of the lungs hinges to the chest wall. I recognized her. It was like looking at a snapshot of her face, though here was only the shadow of her breathing apparatus.

Radiologists trust their machines' power. Dr. Flint had an implicit faith that he could follow the progression of a disease and know a patient's clinical course and fate better than the treating doctors who examined the patient daily. Sometimes seeing the X-ray divulged more information than seeing the patient, but someone has to examine the patient first. As Dr. Flint sat in his darkened reading room, he believed that he could see through patients, that he had special X-ray vision compared to which other doctors were blind.

"He's not getting any better," Dr. Flint would say about Mr. Draper. On another patient's X-ray, he'd remark, "I've never seen anybody's cancer grow as fast as his."

"She's dead," he had judged Judy Langdon, whose eyes he had never glimpsed, whose breaths he had never heard, whose heart he had never palpated beating in his hand as I had, feeling for the point of maximal intensity, the spot just below her left breast where one feels the heart pulsate most strongly.

Radiology is cleaner than other branches of medicine. Radiologists never touch blood or vomitus and never hear throes of pain. They never sniff antiseptic soap masking the stench of diarrhea, or palm sweaty flesh whose pores desperately exude their contents in a last-ditch effort to defend the body. Emergencies are rare in this specialty. The hours are nine to five. Radiology technicians angle, align, and comfort the patients, and snap the pictures. The radiologist only looks at the films after they are developed into negatives. Nothing clings to the crisp plastic sheets. A calm confidence prevails in the radiology suite, removed from nurses and patients.

But radiologists don't always concur. One patient, Mrs. Pisan, had been admitted with searing chest pain that spontaneously diminished. She hadn't suffered a myocardial infarction, or heart attack, but I conducted other tests, looking for a possible dissecting aneurysm—an outpouching of the aorta that spreads by tearing down between the layers of the vessel wall like a rip extending in the seam of a coat. "The radiologists disagree," I informed her one morning, "on whether the CAT scan shows a dissecting aneurysm or not. One says it's there. The other says it isn't."

Mrs. Pisan's hand covered the region of her chest where she had felt pain. She strained to turn to me and spoke. "I know what it shows."

Radiologists have very special tests. For instance, they perform upper gastrointestinal studies. Dr. Flint would have a patient swallow a glass of milkshake spiked with radio-opaque dye. He'd then flick on the TV and follow a gray lump descending the long canal of the esophagus. He'd see the load pushed through the labyrinthine segments of the small intestine. He'd see where the route through the soft tube was obstructed by a bulge, forcing the gray dollop to squeeze through a narrow slit rather than glide along a wide tunnel. Here might be cancer clamped around the hapless bowel like a napkin ring.

Radiologists also perform lower GI studies, in which the dye is introduced rectally. They also squirt dye into the spinal canal to detect blockages along the spinal cord. They have techniques for photographing every organ.

But there were limits to what Dr. Flint could do with his penetrating insight. In his darkened room, he could not participate in deciding what should or would happen to a patient. He was removed from that pressured process.

Adjacent to the Watkins-9 radiology board was Computerized Axial Tomography, or CAT scan room. This was the back room of the radiology suite. The four walls were paneled with metal viewing boxes which encased spotlights. Sheets of glass formed the front of each box. Mounted on the edges of each contraption were clips for inserting radiographic films. When I walked into the room, the boxes were all filled with CAT scans.

Each patient, when CAT-scanned, was laid on a platform which was slowly rolled through a giant electronic "doughnut" that shot and captured X-rays over 360 degrees. A computer then reconstructed a three-dimensional picture of the brain and printed out cross-sectional views on rectangles of film, one-by-two-foot in size, which were subdivided into twelve black squares, each bearing a different perspective. These photos portrayed different slices through the skull. The cuts were horizontal and vertical, front to back and side to side, each picturing the brain a few centimeters up or down, forward or backward, to the right or the left of the adjacent photo. The effect of these many small panels lined across the walls, with patterns of variegated shades illuminated from behind, was that of entering a medieval chapel where light seeps through translucent stained-glass windows. Like a Gothic window, the photographic images were fractionated but they constituted a whole. The room was a black-and-white cathedral of metal ribbing framing these glass sheets. Unfortunately, for many of the abnormalities discovered on this test, including some brain tumors, little treatment exists that is both low risk and effective.

In medieval times, the walls of a cathedral were windows of illuminated pictures showing fragments of the lives of Jesus and various saints, images representing God's presence on earth. In the CAT scan suite, the walls were decorated with images of the human brain, now believed to be the seat of the human soul and man's highest capacities. Though windowless, this room was ethereal and light, a modern sanctuary of the mind.

Stay Tuned

When some patients arrive in the hospital, they immediately clamor for the staff to hook up the television set at the foot of their beds. The Television Hostess, responsible for arranging this, is one of the most frequently paged people in the hospital—often "stat," meaning "immediately."

What would hospitals today be without television? Patients and staff would be more anxious and bored. Television soothes, keeping minds off disease. Patients are reassured by familiar shows. The characters in a sit-com muddle about in the same predicament as when the patient lounged at home.

As I visited patients' rooms during the day, the TV sets were usually on. It was the only time I saw many shows. When programs set in hospitals were aired—"General Hospital" or "St. Elsewhere"—nearly everyone tuned in. As I drew blood from an elderly woman or gave her chemotherapy, I'd find her eyes fixed on the television set, where a young doctor in a white coat stood beside a gray-haired matron's bedside, sampling her blood or injecting a drug. There on the screen were our television portraits. The young doctor seemed less harried than I, unscarred by years of medical training. He was more leisurely, casual, and friendly with his patient than I was, at least on the air, as if he had bumped into her in a grocery store.

I'd have thought patients would turn on anything *but* hospital soaps and sit-coms. Maybe they watched hospital TV because it let them imagine what else went on in a hospital that they couldn't see, like doctors gossiping in the nursing station and nurses complaining.

Even at the bedside of a comatose patient in the Intensive Care Unit, the TV was left on twenty-four hours, barely audible above the sounds of whispering respirator machines and beeping cardiac monitors. The television sound track was believed to provide stimulation for this unconscious patient which might help him if he ever awoke.

Game show contestants won or lost. Wiley Coyote sped off a cliff, realized he was suspended in mid-air, then fell from a fatal height, only to reappear in the next escapade. Cartoon characters survived avalanches, crashes, explosions, and brick walls. The theme song from "The Flintstones" and melodies from frozen foods advertisements jingled in the background as doctors worked.

On hospital soap operas, characters stop by the hospital to say hello to members of the staff. In hospitals I've known this rarely occurs. Hospital TV often has less to do with hospitals, which form the backdrop, and more to do with love and romance, which are rarer in these institutions than is commonly supposed.

Though television isn't realistic, it has the potential to be. For me, working on the ward was like being a character on five television shows at once. I switched from one plot to the serial staged in the room next door. I returned to a story line when I examined a patient, or spotted his chest X-ray or laboratory data. My mind reentered the mystery, chiller, or tragedy. I picked up each where I left off. The character of the doctor delivered the next line to the patient. The next twist in the plot unfolded. Nothing much had happened in the interim while I was away—at least from a medical perspective. To a physician, the important things that happen to a patient revolve around their mutual interaction. A patient's conversation with his family, tears shed, the slow acceptance of disability or death are things a physician excludes from his purview as secondary to the case. The physician decides to start drug A or change to drug B, to operate or to send home. These are the moments and events that the physician deems significant.

As I got to know a patient over days and weeks, I learned more about him or her. I met the family. The patient's clinical course in the hospital rolled on. The patient had ups or downs or suspenseful tests, worsened or improved. Initial leads faltered. Clues faded.

The plots in each of the five shows I was a part of weren't connected except by me. The characters in each story were rarely acquainted. As in episodes of a hospital soap, the scenes bore some resemblance to each other, but the patients and exact themes varied. I was a major character in each. But I acted gentler, firmer, or more paternal depending on the patient. The characters influenced one another. The lines I delivered to a patient affected how he understood his disease and his body, how he felt and replied.

An intern answers myriads of unexpected questions. "Isn't there anything more you can do for my mother? Why did this happen to her? How long does she have to live?" Haunting accusations and prophecies are made. "You're lucky, doc, you're young. You don't know what it's like to be old. Someday you will see." These are quiet moments, seconds when no one else is present but the doctor, and the patient or mother or wife.

Where did my replies come from? From some professional sense, an amalgam of TV and teaching conferences, that congealed, unbeknownst inside me.

Professors of medicine helped perfect my technique, but an intern never has the opportunity to hear one of them pronounce a patient or console a crying family member when visiting hours come to a close at night. A visitor may fear that his loved one may not survive until the morning, that this evening's farewell may be final. What I said often had less to do with formal medical education than what I once said to my grandmother or to a friend, what I read in a novel or saw on a screen.

Sociologists argue that patients play a "sick role." I played the doctor role and sought cues in following my part as much as they did. Sometimes more. I uttered lines that I thought a doctor would utter, acting with the model of the discreet, empathic professional in my mind. When I told a family member a patient was dying, I relied on this model—sympathetic and confident, a stance doctors on television exercise. They're acting. I was playing the real part, but their demeanor and their script prompted mine. What happened to a patient because of my interventions and decisions instructed me and affected my actions and thoughts as I sauntered out of the hospital back to my apartment each night.

My patients couldn't escape home each day. Instead, they watched TV.

Rockette

One afternoon I joined a fellow intern, Ellen Roberts, for a drink after work. We had to plan our outing two and one half weeks in advance to coordinate our on-call schedules. Spending every third night working in the hospital left me with two intervening evenings, one when I was "post-call," and felt drained, and one when I was "pre-call," anxious that the following evening would require me to make tough decisions on little sleep. Emmanuel had recommended going out every third night after being on call and I tried to follow his advice religiously.

We sat in a dark corner of Post Mortem, a local bar.

I had first met Ellen at a meeting during Orientation Week, before internship officially started. She had started the year looking young, almost girlish. Her face appeared more compact now, her skin no longer pink and soft but whitened, and taut against the bones of her cheeks. Her once bouncy black hair was stringy and clung to her head. Her laugh was now edged with a nervous insecurity.

"How are you holding up?" I asked after we were served.

"Overall, I like being an intern."

"Why is that?"

"I like the power."

"The power?"

"Yes. I tell patients and nurses what to do. It's terrible, I suppose. What about you?"

"I find it exhausting."

"I go home wiped out at the end of each day." She lit a cigarette and tapped it into a black ashtray. "I can't do anything.

"I can't stand some of the nurses," she continued. "One or two of them are idiots. I work with one who calls me up at all hours and says, 'Blah blah blah has blah blah blah—what do you want to do about it?' She gives me a difficult time no matter what I do. It's the patients I enjoy—I like them better than the nurses. They're the ones who keep me going."

"Most interns usually don't admit they like patients."

She laughed and tossed back her hair. "Did I ever tell you about my favorite?"

"I don't think so."

"Amelia," she said. "She lived in the hospital for a year and a half."

"What was her story?"

"It's a difficult one, with no beginning, middle, or end. Do you want to hear it anyway?"

"Sure."

"My first day, I was given a list by my resident of patients who were assigned to me. Her name was the first on the sheet. As I walked down the hall, he told me about her. She was sixty-five but she looked in her eighties. An alcoholic for years, she developed hepatitis and eventually complete liver failure. I'll never forget the way she looked. There she was, out cold. Her belly was ballooned out from ascitic fluid accumulated inside, and she looked pregnant." Ellen imitated Amelia's girth, arching her arms out in front of her stomach. Ascitic fluid is protein and glucose that seeps out of obstructed blood vessels, leaking through pores in the vessel's wall as if it were a sieve.

Her white hair was all done up, braided and interwoven with withered flowers. Her liver didn't function, so she couldn't digest protein. If she consumed any, it sent her into hepatic coma, and she'd lie unconscious for twelve hours. Her hand was still clutching three quarters of a pastrami sandwich which she had smeared around her mouth as she had become encephalopathic"—that is, diseased in her brain. "She had gotten confused and it had ended up all over her. I gave her a lactulose enema to help her body excrete the load of protein, and she came back fully alert.

"She constantly tried to cheat on her diet. When I went in that first day, all around her were scattered half-eaten sandwiches. At least once a day she went on food forages, and at least once a week she went into coma.

"She rummaged around the entire hospital to break her diet, stealing from other patients. She'd wander to other wards. I once saw her return with a huge box of chocolates. She had managed to smooth-talk the nurses on another floor to donate it to her. She was very charming."

Ellen swallowed some of her drink.

"She wore a flowery bathrobe a nurse had given her as a present. She loved to 'dress up.' A hospital doesn't have much to dress up with, so she'd drape herself with anything she could get her hands on—old shawls, or those yellow paper disposable isolation gowns nurses wear. I bought her some slippers from Woolworth's with white pom-poms on them. She'd 'do' her hair up with barrette clips. She'd take flowers from other patients' bouquets, sent by their families, and pin them in her hair with the barrettes. She'd borrow makeup and apply lipstick in a wide streak running almost from ear to ear, right across her teeth sometimes. Then she'd sashay down the hall." Ellen flapped her head and hand in imitation.

"Amelia was from Louisiana but had left the South to try to make it in New York City. The South was boring to her; she dreamed of glitter and fancy things and fancy people and getting dressed up. She arrived and somehow got hired on as a Rockette at Radio City. She stayed a Rockette for years. She loved it. Rich men took her out. She probably slept around. She was pretty wild. She told me endless stories about the other girls and Radio City in its glamor days. She was very gossipy. Eventually, she got married, though not to one of her rich boyfriends, and had two kids. Too old for the stage, she stopped kicking and became a housewife. A few years later, her husband died.

"Alone by herself at home, she started to drink, and over the years she couldn't stop. Her two daughters got fed up and moved far away. When she couldn't maintain her apartment, a social worker got involved and had her move to an adult home, where she stayed until she was transferred to the hospital unconscious after a splurge of protein.

"By the time I picked her up, she had been in the hospital for a few months. She'd bleed, losing huge amounts of blood from esophageal varices." These are fragile veins coursing along the esophagus that bloat up with blood backed up from a clogged liver. The vessels occasionally burst.

"Amelia was a big placement problem. I couldn't discharge her anywhere. No nursing home could handle her. Every time she found protein and became stuporous they'd have to haul her back into the Emergency Room. Besides, she'd lose her bed in the nursing home each time and have to be placed again, which can take months. That's the way it works here in this city. So she remained in the hospital, though there was nothing I was actively doing for her other than trying to control her diet, bailing her out with enemas when she managed to outwit me. She lived in the hospital."

I laughed.

"Each week the woman from the Patient Management Office would come around. She read all the charts and approved patients for continued stay or carved them out. Every week, the representative, Linda Poms, an ex-nurse, asked me why Amelia was still here. I'd tell her, and she'd pound the chart with her rubber stamp and scribble something down." The Patient Management Office "carved out" patients when it was suspected that the hospital wouldn't get reimbursed for its expenses by insurance companies or Medicare or Medicaid because the patients weren't being treated aggressively enough to justify continued hospitalization. Ellen told me that Miss Poms hauled around Xeroxed lists of criteria in neat loose-leaf notebooks, but never saw a single patient face to face. "Patient Management" meant hospital budget management. Some patients were discharged because their insurance coverage had run out, though they might need to be readmitted only a short time later. A few extra days now might avert another admission after a few weeks at home. But a chronically ill person admitted twice within a few days was seen as being identical to two different patients by the institution's accounting office. Patients were interchangeable and replaceable. As a hospital administrator once told me, a patient's "marginal cost" to the institution was nil.

"Amelia never did get carved out because she needed to be bailed out every few days. At night, when I was on call she'd visit me. If I had to write up an admission, she'd come by to bum cigarettes and keep me company, telling me her life story. She'd just sit right down in the nurses station. She must have been charming when younger. She thought she still was and could charm anyone into anything. I guess it worked on me.

"No one cared about her except the nurses and me. She'd beg for food and cigarettes. Some of the nurses liked her and bought her barrettes. I used to bring her popcorn—unsalted, of course. A hepatic diet isn't much fun. It's worse than a renal diet and has no protein in it at all. It's basically bread. Can you imagine having to eat only that?

"Amelia would stride into a medical conference that included professors and the chief resident, and say, 'Doctor Ellen'—that's what she called me, 'that's my doctor over there—Doctor Ellen. Could I please borrow a cigarette?' You knew she wasn't ever going to return it. I liked her though. 'Why, the food here is awful today,' she'd complain to me. 'Could you please get me a bag of pretzels from downstairs?' She never had any money, but that went without saying.

"By the time I left she had coded five times but was still on the ward. I was there only for a month. But one morning at breakfast, a few weeks after I left the floor, one of the other interns announced over his coffee, 'Well, Amelia finally boxed.'

" 'You mean she died?' I asked.

" 'Totally dead,' " he said coolly. 'It's probably better for her.'

"I was furious. To the very end, she believed she was going to go home someday. 'I'm going to live with my father in Georgia . . . or with my daughter.' But the previous intern had called them. One daughter was tracked down somewhere in the Midwest and wanted nothing to do with her. Her father had the same response, but Amelia never found out. We never told her."

Ellen looked down at the melting ice cubes in her glass and tapped her cigarette into an accumulated heap of ashes. "One-too-many bites of sandwiches, I guess. Too many chocolates, too much booze . . ." Ellen tilted her glass and watched the dregs of alcohol draw together into a large drop. She shook her head. "Too much."

Old Wounds

I was granted Thanksgiving Day off, at the price of being on call the following day, and traveled with my family to feast at Aunt Irene's. Her Cape Cod colonial house was furnished with cushiony, flowered sofas and exuded a homey calm. This clan, my mother's side of the family, spanned all ages from grandparents to crawling baby cousins.

Within a few minutes of arriving, Aunt Ola, my grandmother's sister, cornered me by the buffet table laid with hors d'oeuvres, a tub of her special chopped liver (brought every year without fail), and a silver tray of celery sticks and slivers of green pepper more to Irene's own taste. Ola was a plump woman, known in the family for "speaking her mind." She preferred to use her full name, Viola, but the rest of the family insisted on calling her Ola. She had long been my favorite aunt—warm, hugging, and the only relative to send birthday and anniversary cards to everyone in the family each year. She kept track of the dates and never failed. She and her husband, Sydney, had flown down from Boston for the holiday. She was wearing bright cherry red stockings with matching shoes and lipstick, and a paisley dress of red, magenta, and blue. From around her neck strings of shiny red plastic beads looped and sloped down onto her breast. She still dyed her hair jet black.

"So you've graduated from medical school, huh? You know," she declared, pointing a silver-ringed finger at my chest, "I never go to doctors."

"Oh?"

"I went to see my doctor. When was it? I forget now . . . the year President Kennedy was elected. What would that make it?"

"1960?"

"I suppose that's right . . . years ago." She flipped her wrist as if to swish away the past. "I don't want to go into the particulars but I had trouble with my equilibrium. People would see me on the street and think I was drunk." She raised her eyebrows to mock the absurdity of such an allegation. She had never confided this story to me before, waiting to tell me until I had finally become a physician. "My doctor sent me to see a specialist in another state, which I did. Well, the specialist thought I had a brain tumor and operated and sent his report back to my own doctor. Before he mailed it, I asked him what it said. He told me, 'It's none of your business.' Do you believe that? The nerve of that man." She nudged me with her elbow and winked. "I wasn't about to take that from him! 'What do you mean, it's none of my business,' I hollered at him. 'It's my brain!'

"I still have the scar here," she said, turning herself around in front of me and bending her neck forward. "Right here," she said, grabbing my index finger, pulling it toward her and placing it on her neck along a faint white scar. I tried to trace the healed line through her hair to see how extensive it was, but her hair had sprouted back too densely.

"My local doctor then sent me to an ear specialist in yet another city, and he did an operation too. Over here," she said, tugging my finger to her temple where the petrous bone above the ear was indented, gouged out. I wouldn't have noticed it if my finger hadn't scooped along the wrinkles flanking her eye. "That time, my local doctor gave me a copy of the first report, sealed with Scotch tape. In the train on the way home," she continued, leaning her head closer to me as if to reveal a secret, "I opened the envelope. The doctor had already broken the seal of tape. And do you know what it said? The specimen the first surgeon had removed had been 'Normal.' On the bottom the bastard had scribbled in "I sure missed the boat on this one." She pointed her finger again. "How do you like that? *That* was twenty years ago," she leaned forward, cupping her hand along the side of her mouth, "before we knew about malpractice."

"Did the second operation help?" I inquired gingerly.

"The problem with my equilibrium disappeared, but I don't think from any operation. To this day, I never trust doctors." She nodded at me as a warning. She had reason to be annoyed.

"Have you seen my two youngest grandchildren lately, by the way?" She had four sons and six grandchildren all together. "Here, let me show you some pictures," she continued. She took two Polaroid snapshots out of her pocketbook.

"They're getting big."

"This one's Judith and that's Lynn." She tapped her fingernail on the film. "Here, I want to show your grandfather."

Her sister, Aunt Pearl, sidled up to me. For years in the family, my grandmother and her two sisters, Ola and Pearl, "weren't talking." The three had preserved their rivalry for decades. I was fond of them all, though. "What was she talking to you about?" Pearl asked.

"An operation many years ago."

"She's never let that one drop," Pearl said. "Of course, I'm

no doctor but I don't think she's been quite the same since."
I didn't comment. "Let me ask you a question. My doctor put
me on three different pills—I think they're for my blood pressure. I don't know much about medications. He has me taking
them at different times of the day. Don't you think I can just
take them all together?" I realized one of the most important
ways in which internship was changing me. People suddenly
perceived me differently—they saw me as a doctor. They asked
my advice, and I was capable of making pronouncements appropriate to that position. I was beginning to think of myself
as a physician, growing more confident, knowing what questions to ask of patients, what answers to give and what ma-
neuvers to perform.

"What are the pills?"

"One's a little white one, the other's yellow, and the third's
pink."

"Do you know their names?"

"No." She didn't feel she should. "But the white one has a
hole in the middle and the yellow one's sort of oblong." I was
equally clueless, unacquainted with the appearance of most of
the medications I prescribe. Pharmacists and nurses do the
dispensing. I only write the orders.

"You should probably follow what your doctor says." I was
behaving with admirable professionalism, supporting the advice of an unknown colleague.

"I have another nephew, he's also a doctor. I think he's in
ENT, though he just does 'E.' The malpractice he has to pay—
you wouldn't believe it. He says he never should have gone
into it and should have been a lawyer instead. My next-door-
neighbor's son, he's in orthopedics. Now, that's where there's
money. He's in practice with three other doctors and is doing
very nicely for himself. He just bought himself a new car. And
I hear he's very good."

———

When Aunt Ola put on her fur hat and coat to leave, she walked up to a younger nephew. Her empty tureen was wedged under her arm. "Here," she said, handing him a rolled-up twenty-dollar bill. "Here's a present." Then she walked up to another nephew, Pearl's grandson, standing beside him. "I'm not giving you anything," she told him, "because your mother never visited me when I was in the hospital back then." It had been twenty years earlier. Pearl, standing behind her, looked up at the light fixture on the ceiling in mock despair. Aunt Ola preserved a vivid and detailed memory and was still a master at guilt. She recalled who had bothered to visit her in the hospital as clearly as she remembered the operation itself.

She turned to me as she was walking out the door. "So, doctor, are you going to send me a bill for your consultation?"

"I'll tell my secretary to mail it out." We both smiled. I wondered if she'd trust at least one doctor more than she had trusted others in the past.

II. Trauma

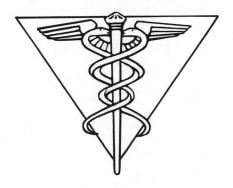

The Biology
of Everyday Life

"**D**o you realize this is probably the only stuff taught in med
school that we'll use outside of work?" A classmate and
I were strolling into a lecture on emergency medicine.

Mr. Ofbar, a medic wearing an unzipped orange wind-
breaker, stood in the front of the auditorium. "I'm going to
talk to you about emergencies," he announced. "I'll show you
cardiopulmonary resuscitation—CPR—and trauma. First, the
basics." He displayed a blood pressure cuff, a hand-pumped
oxygen bag, and a mask.

"Oxygen," he announced earnestly, exhibiting a long and
scraped-up army surplus cannister, "is a clear, odorless, colorless gas that comes in green bottles."

Only in a hospital would oxygen, a constituent of the air,
be described as if it were bottled by Perrier. The natural and
the man-made were naïvely blurred. Above each bed in the
hospital four outlets are installed—for electricity, television,
oxygen, and a vacuum—four essentials of modern life. When

125

tubes are inserted, the vacuum slurps up air or fluid, and oxygen streams out.

Mr. Ofbar's voice hammered on insistently, disallowing any wit or play. All matters were life-and-death. He had no interest in topics, even medical, that weren't of clear immediate and practical value. He didn't care about how the heart functioned, only what techniques would restart it if it failed.

"I'm going to show you slides of injuries seen in emergency rooms," Ofbar said, dimming the lights. He showed photos of bruised, torn, and shredded faces. Accidents had stripped off skin, exposing blood and fat. Spilled acid had singed scalps and scorched pink cheeks. Noses were necrosed or splotched the color of eggplants. The class moaned in revulsion. Never before had I heard these mawkish responses from my medical colleagues. I didn't feel nauseated. I was more struck by the response than the stimulant. My classmates and I had witnessed blood, muck, and gore. While dissecting a corpse, I had severed limbs and hacked open ribs, sawed through a pelvic bone, and drilled through a skull. I had scooped up a watery brain in my hands as it slopped halfway out of its case. I had assisted in grueling surgical procedures, yanking at muscles and layers of fat. So had the others. But this squeamishness was new. Deformed limbs or kidneys hadn't nauseated the class; these mauled faces did.

Certainly I had felt disgusted by other things in the past. The first time was when I attended my first surgical procedure. Both the nurse and the surgeon forewarned me that I might start feeling ill, and that I could just step to the corner or out of the room if I chose.

"Not me," I had thought. After all, I had dissected a fetal pig and had already studied biology.

The first forty minutes had proceeded smoothly. I towered over a nurse who was also observing, and witnessed an "insider's" view of the action. But, as a random piece of bowel was sliced, a bleeding vessel was cauterized with the metal tip of an electric knife, toasting the leaking vein to seal it off. A blue whiff of smoke wafted up from the burning tissue and curled into my nostrils.

The next thing I knew, a nurse was assisting me out of the darkened room into the bright and spacious hallway. She handed me over to a cordial nurse well acquainted with these exigencies, who led me to the lounge next door. There she saw to it that I lay down on the floor with my feet propped up on a chair and my head hard against cold linoleum tiling. She handed me a paper cup of orange juice to sip. Some doctor I was going to make!

Within a few minutes, though, the queasiness passed and I got to my feet.

"You want to go back in?" the nurse asked, surprised.

My head no longer spun. "Sure."

I resumed my position observing fat, flesh, and blood. This conglomeration wasn't soup, I told myself, but was anatomy. I tried to concentrate on how a surgeon must look at it. I began to see it only as "tissue" and not as something human. This yellow and red pulsating mass kept my body running and was me. Drapes concealed the arms and legs, the face, and the rest of the body. A nimble nurse slid a table of instruments over to the incision site so that it seemed we were digging a hole into the table. The arrangements bore little resemblance to an open human dissection, making it more tolerable. I told myself that this should not disgust me.

Once that was said, I was less offended. I allowed myself to see the parts, each working, performing its separate job, and not be overcome by the ugliness of the whole.

I felt queasy another time, after having my blood drawn as part of a routine checkup. I watched with fascination as the dark red liquid shot into a glass vacuum tube. I had to lie down on the black leather examining table for several minutes to regain my balance. But this experience didn't flatten me as much as that first day in the OR.

The only other time I ever felt faint was when I broke my wrist. I had fallen and landed on my left hand. The wrist and hand quickly swelled up, the skin rising pale and puffy. I no longer recognized this soft, round, fleshy, painful hand. I had to lie down on the ground.

When I saw my own blood squirting out or layers of a body that shouldn't have been exposed, my body acted as if it was injured and tried to lie down quickly. My body thought it shouldn't be going anywhere in that condition. To traipse around might risk having brain cells gasping for air. The best response was to faint, ensuring a peak supply of blood to my head. Fainting was a practical, though not specific, reaction, an adaptive biological response.

The first day of medical school, I began dissecting a cadaver in a gross anatomy course. "If any of you start to feel ill," Dr. Toller warned the class, "just step out of the room." I remembered my experience in the operating room a few years earlier. Several students, including one of my team members, Katherine, had to excuse herself. Not I.

People say, "I wanted to be a doctor but couldn't stand the sight of blood." I couldn't either initally. But after only three exposures, my neurological system was desensitized and adapted. A weak stomach can be overcome. By the time Dr. Ofbar displayed these mutilated faces in class, I had told myself that this was interesting, seeing what human beings looked like. Medical training had distanced me from a visceral reaction.

Built into the brain is a specialized center responsible for inspecting faces—analyzing daily masks. Research has shown that primates as well as humans have a significant portion of their craniums committed to this crucial social task of sorting through subtle differences in faces. My emotions are strongly tied to these centers, expert at differentiating between my father and my uncle, for instance, and reading in a friend's face nuanced clues of distress, rage, or warmth.

How many faces do I know? Hundreds? Thousands? I recently bumped unexpectedly into an old acquaintance on the street. We both stopped short and searched each other's face, but were unable to remember each other's name. The linguistic portion of my brain lagged behind the facial recognition center in retrieving her name. We both continued in our tracks, then halted, glanced over our shoulders, and confronted each other.

"Don't I know you?"

Only seconds later did her name come to my tongue, with uncertainty.

". . . Emily?"

". . . Robert . . . Bob?" She tried to remember which name I preferred or which she used to call me.

The brain even disregards changes that occur with time and recognizes constant features. When Proust returned to a salon after many years' absence and spied former friends, at first he thought they were wearing gray wigs, but then realized they'd only aged. His brain performed complex adjustments. The brain places great stock in defining people by their faces. Sensitive distinctions are crucial to the social events of love and war that serve as the scenes of natural selection.

A comparable kidney recognition center doesn't exist, since the human brain as it evolved didn't have to identify kidneys. Cosmetic facial damage violated our cultural and biological senses of beauty. There seemed to be an innate biology of aesthetics. It follows from Darwin's theory of the survival of the fittest, that an organism identifies the most attractive members of the opposite sex for pursuit and mating. A portion of the brain screens for beauty, though what particular features excite these neurons may vary among different cultures and individuals. Courting and falling in love involve complex physiological processes. Thus, the brain intrinsically shuns what is grotesque, sensing that we should avoid diseased faces around which contagion may lurk.

The experiences of both affection and disdain, the latter of which underlies much prejudice, are encoded by the same biological mechanisms—neuronal pathways and chemical transmitters. Sitting in the lecture hall, I realized that strong visceral responses are evoked by seeing injured faces. For many in the class, a biological offense occurred. These slides sickened the substantial hunk of brain that spots the familiar through the maimed.

But medical education had numbed this reaction in others of us. I observed these responses but remained silent and unmoved. When this class was over, I headed off to the next.

Hospital Codes

"Mr. Otis has just been pronounced," a nurse, Donna, croaked into the phone hanging on the Emergency Room wall. She banged the black receiver down on its hook. Those were her only words.

His story was quite ordinary; his fate might await anyone. Conscious half an hour earlier when he arrived at the Emergency Room, his heart had stopped. The two nurses present at the time took up their positions. Alan, a male nurse, started performing cardiopulmonary massage (CPR), pumping on the patient's chest in a steady rhythm. He was regularly assigned to the Emergency Room, and was geared for immediate crises. Anne-Marie, a nurse in her early twenties, yanked the special red knob on the wall.

Throughout every hallway in the entire hospital, from every loudspeaker, the call in process was immediately chanted: *Code Six: Emergency Room . . . Code Six: Emergency Room.* Medical personnel understand what a "Code 6" is. But most patients were unaware of the call's meaning. To be reminded on the PA system that people die in this building each day would cause them unnecessary distress.

For Mr. Otis, residents, interns, and medical students, lab technicians and a priest dropped their work and hurried downstairs into a cubicle in the ER. Nineteen people showed up, including Emmanuel, Walt, a surgeon named Dr. Yamamoto, a resident named Laura Wyckoff, a priest, Anne-Marie, Alan, and Donna, who ran down from the Medical Intensive Care Unit, where she worked. Some stragglers stood on the sidelines, out of the way, and watched the spectacle, occasionally running errands to deliver specimens of blood or fetch additional supplies.

By the time most of us got there, "the code," as the attempted rescue is called, was well under way. Dr. Yamamoto tended the head, squeezing an oxygen bag with mechanical precision. Donna hung up bulging bags of fluid on poles and ran clear plastic tubing over to the body. Yellow caps from hypodermic needles were cast onto the edges of the stretcher where Mr. Otis lay. In the fluorescent light, bits of paper ripped from alcohol pads glinted. Spurts of blood welled into the sheets.

I took Alan's place doing the CPR. I stepped up onto a stool and pushed heavily down upon the body, reminded not to bend my elbows while pumping. I pressed down rhythmically, fierce but patient.

"Who's running this code?" Dr. Wyckoff, the resident, yelled out.

"A nurse is," Alan yelped.

"Where's the EKG machine?" she demanded, sizing up the ammunition supply with a hard eye. "I want a blood gas sent." Donna drew a sample of arterial blood so that the amount of oxygen and carbon dioxide percolating through it could be measured, to assess how effectively Mr. Otis's lungs aerated his body.

"Let's give him an amp of epinephrine," Dr. Wyckoff declared, manning the EKG machine, which was built into a wheeled cart and hooked up to the man's still-warm limbs. It spewed forth tape on which the needle had traced a fluttery line representing either ventricular fibrillation or background noise. Dr. Wyckoff had witnessed many such battles, and maintained the poise of a military strategist in the thick of heavy fighting.

New faces showed at the periphery as staff members flung the curtain aside. The scene was chaotic, conversations fragmented, yet the single goal of reviving Mr. Otis's body drew all our frantic efforts like a vortex.

Dr. Yamamoto slid a sickle-shaped tube into the patient's throat to prop the mouth open for the flow of air. Chomping without pause on the piece of gum in his mouth, Dr. Yamamoto carefully aligned the neck of the tube and taped it to the patient's slack lips.

Anne-Marie gripped a clipboard and addressed the crowd. "Does anyone know what his name is?" Donna joined us, having just conversed with the patient's wife in the hallway, gathered details about him. Only now did a picture of our patient begin to emerge. Aged fifty-nine, Mr. Otis had a history of high blood pressure and angina pectoris (that is, chest pain due to lack of oxygen in the muscle of his heart). An hour before, he'd been standing in his bathroom at home when pain gripped his chest. His wife had eased him down onto the floor and called the ambulance. Earlier that afternoon he had been fine, working in his garden. Now, he might never leave the ER alive.

"Stop compressions," Dr. Wyckoff ordered. I stood aside. The team was silent. The tape ticked on as all eyes squinted at the bumpy line on the paper.

"I don't feel a femoral pulse," Alan declared from beside me.

"Start compressions," Laura cried. "I want a Doppler machine." All manned their stations. I again began to pump. My palm flattened on his chest every second with the wet squish of sweaty skin. A dry oxygen bag heaved with a raspy voice. More blood samples were hurried down to the blood gas lab.

Anne-Marie soothed the skin on his neck, feeling for the throb of life. "He has no carotid pulse," she intoned as if to herself. "But I feel a femoral pulse with the compressions."

"He has no blood pressure," Alan shouted from behind.

"Give him calcium," came Dr. Wyckoff's voice. The team worked on, occasionally halting compressions and injecting medications, but his heart never roused.

"Let's buzz him," she commanded. I was handed two plastic paddles. I positioned them on his chest.

"All stand clear," Alan shouted.

"We're shocking him," Donna announced. Everyone backed off, leaving me alone with the patient and megavolts of current. I arched my arms up over the body so as not to ground myself on his skin. My thumbs tautened in the air above the red plastic buttons on each electrode, ready to crack lightning into the body. The room held its breath.

"Now?" I asked, frightened.

"Go ahead," Laura instructed calmly. I jabbed the buttons with my thumbs. The body jerked up tensely and then flopped back down onto the stretcher. I felt stunned, as if the current had passed through my own moist palms and seared my heart.

"Resume contractions," I heard. I felt my body mechanically levering up and down over his. Still no pulse or blood pressure. On the EKG machine's roll of graph paper, a timorous needle inked a tall hump each time my palms pressed down on his chest. I squinted to detect any ripples of electrical activity following each of these big waves.

Laura punctured the wall of his chest between two ribs with a wide-bore needle, aiming toward his heart to see whether the sack surrounding the heart—the pericardium—had ballooned out with blood, hampering the heart itself from filling. She suctioned out blood, which gurgled up into a horse-sized syringe. It turned out that the blood was from inside the heart, not outside, and wasn't preventing the cardiac chambers from being filled.

"Stop compressions," Laura instructed. Silence fell. The soft whirr of the EKG machine was the only sound we heard.

She breathed in air and courage. "We've given it an hour," she announced. "Let's call the code."

Quietly, hands withdrew from the clutter on the table. The dial on the EKG machine clicked several times as Laura turned it to the OFF position. Discarded syringes cluttered the bed. Squares of bloodstained gauze pads littered the sheets and floor. I slowly helped gather up the flotsam and jetsam. Donna went over to the phone. Glued to the receiver was a yellow sticker that read *Organ Donor Hotline,* and provided a phone number—a reminder to consider salvaging healthy organs from the dead. Trauma victims make ideal donors, since their uninjured organs are presumably disease free. Yet none of us mentioned the possibility of harvesting organs from Mr. Otis. I heard Donna's voice on the phone informing the hospital administration that Mr. Otis had been pronounced. She came the closest to admitting that anything had transpired.

A rotund priest slipped in silently from the back, having followed his cue countless times before. Anne-Marie straightened up from bending over the floor, where she was collecting discarded wrappings. "Well, we did what we could do," she chirped. "Now it's your turn." He went to the head of the table, placed his fingers over the man's wide eyelids, and slipped out again.

"Is this his sweater?" Anne-Marie shouted, holding up a blue pullover as if at an auction. No one knew.

"I'll tell the wife," Laura said and sighed.

Mrs. Otis was pacing in the hallway around the pay phone, where she had been calling friends and relatives in tears. Crumpled tissues had accumulated around the phone. Laura sat down with her beside a black leather examining table in an empty cubicle across the hall and told her what had happened.

Four of us—Alan, Anne-Marie, Donna, and I—rolled him over to wrap a white plastic sheet around the body. His limp arms dangled from the bed. I lifted one of them up, holding his meaty palm in mine as if shaking hands.

"I didn't get to see the reports on two of the three blood gases," Donna reflected, now that the dark clouds had cleared.

She strung the two feet together at the ankles with rope. "Why are you tying him up?" I asked.

"For transport," she answered. The transport personnel would have to shoulder the corpse out.

"I haven't done this in a while," Anne-Marie chatted, as she lifted the feet up and pulled the plastic behind them again, adjusting the wrapping on the package.

"We do this all the time upstairs in the MICU," answered Donna. She pronounced it "mick-you."

Anne-Marie smoothed out the sheet neatly over the corpse and tucked in the edges. "Where are the things he came in with?" she asked.

"He didn't have any," Donna answered, tying more knots around the ankles.

"No, here are his underwear and pants," Anne-Marie proclaimed. She picked up the bag containing the clothes. "Well, here are his worldly possessions," she whispered as she plopped the loose parcel of clothes down against the wall.

Alan whisked out catheters from the veins in the patient's

arms. I sheared off the tape around a catheter that had been inserted into his heart.

"Just pull it?" I asked. Another dumb question.

"Yup," Alan answered. He slipped a piece of gauze into my hand to swab any fresh blood, but the catheter slid out with no blood at all.

Mr. Otis's eyelids floated open, revealing thin watery slivers of white at each eye. Alan quickly reshut them. I pulled the tape from the thick unshaven flesh and slid the tracheal tube out of his mouth.

Alan tried removing the chain of dogtags from around Mr. Otis's neck. He attempted to pull it over the head but it fit too tightly. He searched for a clasp, but the chain appeared to form a continuous circle without break. He pulled the chain over the chin, and then over the moist nose. The links scraped the loose skin and caught on the eyelids, pulling them open—completely this time—to reveal two round dark eyes in the middle of their white fields, gazing straight out.

The patient was wearing two rings. Alan twisted a gaudy one off the plump finger which it had gripped for years. He reached across the nude corpse for the other, a simple wedding ring.

Donna interrupted. "Sometimes wives like to keep wedding rings, and sometimes they like to have them go with them. I've seen it both ways." Alan wrapped white masking tape around the finger, securing the ring.

Anne-Marie took three cards out of a package, each with a hole punched in it, through which a string was threaded. "Here, fill these out," she said, handing them to me. One read, "Attach to Outside," one, "Attach to Personal Effects Bag," and the third, "Attach to Big Toe." I inscribed the patient's name on each and gave the last of these to Donna, who tied the string around a stubby toe that protruded from the plastic.

"He needs a pillow," Anne-Marie decided. But none of us bothered to fetch one.

We wheeled the stretcher into a private room for Mrs. Otis to see, as she had requested. I closed the door and drifted away. I felt helpless, connected with what had happened, but now with nothing left to do about it.

I floated into the cramped doctor's office next door. Laura sat at a desk, before an empty green blotter. She glanced up at me and then turned back to face the wall. I sank into a swivel chair at the far end of the room. A secretary from the front desk appeared in the doorway and said to Laura, "There's a crowd out there in the waiting room, doctor. Your other appointments are all getting impatient." They had been stalled for an extra half hour.

Laura appeared distracted. "When a code is run, it takes a while to see everybody else."

Two thick folders of Mr. Otis's old medical records sat on the desk in front of me. The edges of their pages, yellow, white, and pink, were crushed from frequent handling. Now they would be filed away and forgotten.

An older administrative nurse hobbled up to my desk, perusing a form in her hand which she shoved at me. "Mr. Otis needs a short admission form filled out," she announced. I looked up at her quizzically from over the stacks of old records. Though the patient was no longer alive, he still had to be admitted to the hospital. She read the puzzlement in my eyes. "Officially, patients never die in the Emergency Room," she explained. "They have to be listed as dying in an ICU"—the facility best equipped for monitoring cardiac arrests.

After she'd left, the phrases welled up in my dazed mind. Mr. Otis hadn't died, he had just "been pronounced," and it hadn't happened in the Emergency Room because such things aren't allowed to happen there.

I took a deep breath, stood up, and walked slowly over to the box containing the charts of patients waiting to be seen. I picked up the manila folder on the top of the pile. Slim and new with the edges still crisp, it had the light feel of a simple medical problem, the kind that can be solved. I wandered out to meet my next patient.

Guts

Luis Fontana was triaged to the trauma section of the Emergency Room. A sixteen-year-old Hispanic, he had tried to kill himself by slashing his stomach in a long slit from one flank to the other. The wound was superficial, never piercing through protective layers of muscle. The wound opened a wide set of lips on his abdomen. He told the triage nurse who had interviewed him when he arrived in the ER that his girlfriend of five months had left him. His parents were separated, and his family poor. His parents, who had been unmarried, had fought incessantly at home. I learned that he had no one to talk to. Even if he had, he wouldn't have known quite what to say. He wanted to end it all, to escape.

What he ended up with was me. I sewed the skin back up across his belly, squirting local anesthetic in the track of my needle and thread. I used the standard painkiller—lidocaine —a short-acting drug, the dulling strength of which wore off quickly. The gash pained him. My first sutures stung him. He bolted up and babbled in Spanish, presumably that he wanted to be left alone and let out.

140

"You have to get stitches, Luis," I told him. "The sooner you cooperate, the sooner it'll be done."

He jabbered on.

"Lie down," I commanded him in English in my most forceful tone. He understood. Behind me stood two imposing policemen, hovering like giant shadows, their hands on their hips. When I gave Luis this command, one of the cops nodded at him, reinforcing my words. Enraged, Luis switched his glare from me to the policemen and then resigned himself to falling back down under the pull and tug of my white silk sutures as I proceeded to sew him up further.

I had been taught the various styles of knots used by surgeons, but my teachers had little time or patience to watch me practice while standing in the operating room with patients under closely monitored general anesthesia. Trainees were advised to improve their technique by sewing up the peels of fresh oranges, said to have the same tough resistance to being pierced as human skin.

Luis required almost one and a half feet of minuscule weave, and I was required to perfect my skill, whether either of us liked it or not. I learned to prick the flap of skin close enough to the edge so that the needle didn't need to dig through too many layers of epidermis, yet far enough away that the skin didn't break, destroying the hole.

I tried three surgical stitches of one type, experimented with five of another, ten of the loop-the-loop variety, and fifteen in which the silk thread is cut and tied after each pass of the needle. The procedure probably took two hours, though it seemed longer to me, and, I suspect, even more interminable to him.

Once Luis had resigned himself to my suturing, the two cops backed away toward the doorway and began to chat.

"How many commendations do you need to get three stars?" one asked the other.

"Four. With five, you go over to silver."

"No, with five you get a gold. The fourth is silver. Three you get a bronze."

"What I was trying to figure out was—if you go over seven, do you start all over?"

"No, you add a bronze."

"Why not add another gold? I think that'd be better."

Luis cursed.

I began to like Luis as I sewed him up. When I was finally done, I straightened up, stretching my back, and inspected his abdomen, my work of art. Some stitches were woven close together, others were spread out more evenly and farther apart. The rough black line zigzagged in patches. I had never sutured to this extent and felt proud of my handicraft, more confident in my manual dexterity as a physician.

I would only have to write a sentence or two on his ER sheet. My job was simply putting him back together by knitting together opposing flaps of skin. When I was finished, Luis was wheeled off, and taken to the Psychiatry area, where he would be examined to determine whether a psychiatric hospitalization would help put him back together in other ways. Solving these other problems would take much longer to do.

III. Neurons

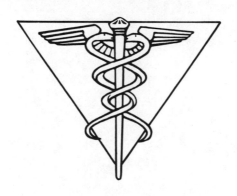

Without Words

W hile in medical school, I wondered what I would be missing by becoming a doctor. I decided to sit in on a class in comparative literature taught by Professor Paul deMan, a leading literary critic in the Graduate School at Yale, where I was then a student. Each week, as the late afternoon light filtered through the classroom's Gothic windows overlooking the "Old Campus," deMan argued the primacy of language in understanding works of literature. No historical, psychological, or sociological data were relevant to the interpretation of any work. Literature was about language, not about anything else in the world. Theories that touched on anything outside the piece of literature were rejected (Marx, deMan once decried, was "a mere aesthetician"). All actual human experience was implicitly irrelevant to the reading of these texts. In the evenings, deMan's graduate students sat around a local bar, The Anchor, and debated his theories.

The following year, during internship, I worked on a neurology ward. There, I met Marian Czesnefsky. Better than anyone I had ever known, she answered the argument voiced in that cloistered classroom. Implicitly, to deMan, human interactions consisted fundamentally of an interchange of words. Language and literature alone were what mattered most in human affairs. Marian taught me something else.

She was a short, elderly woman who had been picked up by the police at 4:00 A.M. wandering through the streets in her nightgown. She knew neither her name nor her address and had no identification on her. When asked questions, she'd just nod along.

"What's your name?" a neurology resident would bark into her ear. With each failure to respond, he'd shoot the question at her more loudly, as if she were deaf rather than neurologically impaired.

"My name," she'd repeat in a firm tone, as if delivering a definitive answer. She seemed to be in perfect health, and looked in her mid-seventies. Since her neurological status was otherwise intact, it was concluded that she was aphasic and had sustained a small stroke in areas of her brain that are responsible for language.

She was now a patient on the ward, but there was little that could be done for her. Her laboratory test results printed in compact boxes on computer paper showed that her blood cell counts, her thyroid function studies, her electrolytes—or salts in the blood—and other measurements were all normal. She seemed to have suffered from either Alzheimer's disease or, what might be more likely since she had apparently managed to function adequately until now, a multi-infarct dementia.

She was started on one aspirin tablet a day to dilute her blood slightly in order to prevent further strokes. But no effective therapy reverses strokes, and there was nowhere to send her. What does one do with a charming old lady, a LOLNAD (standard medical jargon for "a little old lady in no acute distress") whose major problem is that she can't think of the words she wants to use? She knew how to behave appropriately. She'd bow and wave cheerfully to everyone who walked by. She was the only patient on, the ward to make her own bed each morning. She helped the nurses at night, tying rubber bands onto laboratory order slips. Though speechless, she'd entertain other patients who needed to sit with someone. She wandered up and down the halls in a hospital-supplied bath-robe wrapped almost double around her frail but firm body, her hands clasped behind her back as she paraded.

After she'd been in the hospital for three days, she recovered a handful of words. But the neurologists, or "Neurons" as they were nicknamed by doctors in other specialties, thought she wouldn't progress much further. When tested for self-care com-petency, she displayed difficulty lighting a stove, cooking a hard-boiled egg, balancing a checkbook, and performing other essential domestic tasks. She wasn't going to get much further with her English or, more importantly, with what is called in medicine her "disposition." This term referred to the issue of where I was going to deposit or "dispo" her eventually, how I was going to get her off my hands.

Patients were admitted every day. They had to be "worked up" and sent off, or "dispo'ed," as efficiently as possible. It was necessary to discharge them to their homes or to relatives, to nursing homes or other hospitals, or to "turf" them to a different medical specialty in the same institution, such as cardiology or psychiatry. If the other discipline accepted them only briefly, and then returned them to their original ward, they were said to "bounce back." The problem of disposition would then be faced anew. If patients didn't turn over rapidly, empty beds would never be available for new patients. As soon as a patient was admitted, I was told to begin to think about where to send him or her after we had completed the necessary medical procedures.

My newly arrived patient, though she had become the ward

mascot, had no disposition. With no name, address, social security number, or known source of income or support, the hospital would be unable to send her anywhere. Government agencies would refuse to accept her. To bureaucracies, she simply wouldn't exist, and in the mind of my resident, this was now her biggest problem. She could be here for months or years, even for life.

"Someone has to figure out her story," my resident announced one morning on rounds. "Whoever does deserves special recognition." My interest was piqued. Not that my appetite hadn't been whetted beforehand. I was as much taken by this woman's charisma and appearance as I was by the philosophical questions she presented as to the role of language and the encoding of speech in a few fleshy bulges of the left hemisphere of the brain. I volunteered for the job.

I started by spending several hours with her. We clearly liked each other. I began to realize that she understood the gist of my questions, but responded to them poorly. There was impairment in Broca's and, to a lesser degree, Wernicke's area of the brain. Broca's area, located roughly in front of the left ear on most right-handed people (and above the right ear in some left-handers), is responsible for linguistic expression. Wernicke, a German neurologist, discovered that a few shiny lumps of brain just behind Broca's area are responsible for understanding speech.

I asked my patient all about the neighborhood where she had been found, giving her an opportunity to respond with whatever gestures or responses she could. One day, she started rotating her shoulders and flipping her elbows, and I realized that she was imitating swinging a baseball bat. Though initially perplexed, I asked if she was trying to tell me that she lived near the baseball stadium. Her eyes lit up. I had scored a point. I dragged out a city map and read aloud a number of street names surrounding the ballpark. At some, her face brightened.

A few words began to dribble back to her. She would come up to me in the hall, shaking her fist when she was angry. "You . . . you . . . you . . . you . . ." she'd declare, as if interspersing the pronoun with a silent insult. Her small fist shook, as she flexed her wrist awkwardly. Unable to think of the epithets she wanted to hurl at me, she'd just repeat "you" and jitter her fist in a half-mocking threat.

One morning, answering a question about her name, she managed to articulate the syllables "Chez-nef-sky." She seemed as startled as I was, and her eyes betrayed a shock of self-recognition. Grasping this clue, I eagerly searched the telephone directory, but in vain. No such name was listed.

Frustrated by my inability to identify her, I left the hospital one afternoon to drive around her presumed neighborhood. I talked to people in the street, and passing a senior citizen center, inquired within. A janitor who doubled as a first aid attendant directed me to the apartment of Sissy Miserbach. A matriarchal yenta, she sat in the middle of a cramped apartment stuffed with the mementos of an ebbing life. She knew everybody's business at the center, but she didn't recognize my patient's description.

Back at the hospital, my patient's spirits were beginning to sag. "Home . . . home," she whispered to herself, staring out mournfully at the snowy streets beneath her sealed, insulated window. For her, the unopenable glass might as well have been metal bars. Somewhere out there, I thought, was her home— but where? I'd try to console her, to tell her I couldn't obtain her address. I don't know if she comprehended my dilemma, if she sensed that she had suffered a neurological loss, that her language was impaired, that I wanted to send her home, but that she might never be able to live independently in her own apartment again. She shook her fist more regularly, that gesture communicating what she would have said in paragraphs if she could have spoken. She held her head high, in embittered dignity. She was tough, but the imprisoning banality of the hospital was taking its toll.

I wondered what her first language was, based on the Central or Eastern European accent with which she uttered her handful of words.

"German?" I asked her. She revealed no sign of recognition.

"Russian?" She vaguely shook her head.

"Czech?" Her head said no in emphatic disdain.

"Polish?" Her face broke out into energetic wrinkles and she pointed to my lips with a smile.

Posted in the nursing station was a list of translators—mostly hospital employees, their families, and friends who happened to speak a second language. Under "Spanish" was a long list of names, and a shorter list under "French." A radiologist spoke Japanese, and a laboratory researcher was fluent in German. One translator each was listed for Hindi, Persian, Korean, and Polish, as well as for several others.

The Polish translator, a filmmaker, greeted the patient in his own language, and she nodded. I posed questions to translate. He was a patient man; but her native tongue was preserved only marginally more than her English.

I suspected that she had a multi-infarct dementia caused by tiny blood clots showering the vasculature of the brain and blocking off the tiny arterioles that supply blood and oxygen throughout this organ. The hospital had installed a special brain-imaging device which was being researched for its use in differentiating between multi-infarct dementia and Alzheimer's disease. A radioactive substance is injected into the patient, and the machine traces the routes of arteries pulsing through the brain. Areas that are suffused inadequately appear blank.

My resident decided that she would be tested, and one afternoon, I strolled with her over to the radiology lab. In the waiting room, she was brought a radioactive dye stored in a sealed lead vial. I sat with her there as she was injected with its contents. She looked at me nervously, trusting the test because of my presence. She was led into a room and her body was secured into a white machine with a special metal band encircling her head. The machine looked like the contraption in the middle of a planetarium that projects the lights of stars onto the ceiling. Once she was strapped in, the device pivoted around its center in all directions, tilting her up and down and rotating her on its axis. The action, similar to an amusement park ride, bewildered her. She was reassured spotting me behind a glass control booth as she moved by.

The test results were equivocal, and didn't alter the treatment. Perhaps partly because of the mounting stress, however, slight improvement followed.

One morning she spoke a name.

"Gert O'Casey."

I found the name in the city directory, and phoned. Gert O'Casey turned out to be a close friend, and gave me some facts about the patient. Her name was Marian Czesnefsky, but she had two names: one from the old country, one for the bureaucrats here in the New World. She had been listed in the phone book all along, under the name Mary Simmons. Retired for fifteen years, she had worked for decades as a seamstress. Gert and Marian had evolved a delicate mutual dependence. Marian could walk well but, I discovered, had suffered from impaired manual dexterity for several years. Gert tottered badly even when using a heavy cane, but she was younger and could cook. Marian did the grocery shopping. Gert was their hands and Marian their feet. But Mrs. O'Casey was being admitted to the hospital for surgery on her leg, the outcome of which was uncertain. Both of their futures were now in doubt.

Armed with knowledge of our patient's identity, I applied for government benefits on her behalf, but was informed that processing and approval could take weeks, even months.

Marian felt abandoned by the rest of the staff. Nurses had to give most of their time to patients who required closer and more acute care, leaving her more to herself. I became her only source of possible salvation. She would clench my arm with her fine wrinkled hands. "Home . . . home," she would plead. A helpless little girl returned from days back in Cracow at the dawn of the century and swam in a well of tears. "Home" might still lie somewhere in Eastern Europe.

Within two weeks, my rotation on the ward drew to a close. Following a hardened medical tradition, the house staff and medical students would be moving on, abandoning the patients whom they had come to know, and in some instances, love. New staff would take over and start from the beginning. For some patients, this change in healers passes off smoothly. But for patients such as Marian, the transition confuses and disrupts.

On the afternoon of my last day, I paid her my final visit. I assumed it would be the last time I would ever see her.

She smiled as I walked into her room. I didn't know if she'd understand what I had to tell her. I, her one hope left in the world, was now deserting her too. "Things will be okay," I told her wistfully. "We're working on getting you out of here." But I couldn't say where to. "I have hope for you. Another doctor will be taking over who is very good." I didn't know who he was, or whether he would interact with her more than marginally. In his mind, she might be instantly labeled as "awaiting discharge," a curse for any hospital inpatient, who might then receive only minimum attention from doctors and nurses caring for needier patients.

Marian cried. I noticed that her gray hair was no longer neatly pulled back; straying wisps floated about her head. Her room was lined with plants and bouquets of faded flowers that she had collected from the rooms of patients being discharged. Perhaps in her mind these plants symbolized the fact that others had been liberated and that she might too, one day.

I saw Marian once after that. Two months after I left her in the hospital, she was accepted into a small nursing home in an affluent residential area. I visited her there one cold day in December, just before Christmas.

The institution occupied a maroon brick building in a quiet neighborhood. Brown branches of ivy clung to its walls like veins. A sharp wind rustled through half-barren trees and scraped frail leaves along the sidewalk.

As I approached her in the lobby, confusion clouded her face. But as we began to talk, a glimmer of recognition appeared in her eyes. She remembered me after hearing my voice.

The staff escorted us into a visitors lounge. As we sat, sunlight brightened the wrinkles of her pale face and illuminated her hair. She wore light pink pants, doubled over at the waist and cuffed at the legs. A silver ring graced her hand, although a metal stud protruded from it where a jeweled stone, now lost, had once sat.

I was curious how much language she had recovered. I pointed to my shoe and asked if she knew the word for it. "It's a . . . a . . . a . . . it's a big one," she stumbled out, referring to my size 10 Wallabees.

I pointed to my watch. "Do you know what this is called?" She smiled back blankly. She hadn't understood. "What is the *name* for this?" I inquired.

"Czesnefsky!" she responded, pleased.

"What is it?" I asked again, tapping my watch band.

"It is a . . . a . . . I have one too," she announced and

slowly folded back her sleeve, reaching for a bracelet on her wrist. She unclasped it to display it with pride. "Here," she said. "Here," pointing with a quivering finger to the inside of the bracelet as if an inscription were to be found. But there was no writing there, at least not any longer. Nor had she noticed it was gone. The memory of words was all she had now in place of words that were themselves lost.

"Is this your home?" I asked gently.

"My home?" she repeated, as if asking herself what the words meant.

"Where do you live?"

"Mine . . ." She sputtered the name of the city.

"Where in the city?" I inquired.

"I live . . . right on the . . . the . . ." She shuttled her hand back and forth in the air in front of her as if to signify a street. "Here is me," she proclaimed, pointing to the seam on the plastic couch cushion on which she sat. "And there," she said, gesturing to the empty center of the room in a shaky voice. "There is the chu . . . the church." She still didn't know the word "street" or the name of the street where her apartment had been located.

"Is this where you live?"

"We sleep, we eat . . . All of us, we . . ." She drew a circle with her hand in front of her as if motioning to a crowd of people filling the room. She couldn't say that they "lived" there, what kind of place it was or its name.

The staff informed me that Marian had run away from the institution several times. The first time, she disappeared for three days. Nearby hospitals were called daily to see if she had been brought in, and ads were run in the city papers, but to no avail. She eventually was found wandering in her old neighborhood, which she had somehow discovered. To this day, no one knows where she spent those three nights, and she is unable to say. She has escaped other times since and has always returned to the vicinity of her old street. She apparently roams through the neighborhood until she comes across a subway and then navigates her way beneath the streets, though she can't communicate her address. An ID bracelet had now been buckled around her wrist, carrying a small square plastic box. Whenever she approaches the main entrance of the nursing home, the gadget sets off an electronic alarm. A nurse rushes to the vestibule where Marian stands, confused by the shrill noise around her.

"I like my . . . my things," she confided. "All I have is my . . . my . . ." Words again failed her. She reached up and fingered her hair. She couldn't elaborate further on the thought in her head, but her gesture suggested that her hair, her body were her sole remaining possessions.

"Where's Gert?" I asked. Her face remained blank. "Remember Gert?"

"Gert," she repeated. A flash of recognition jarred her face. She remembered the name but could say nothing else.

Every few minutes as she sat with her legs crossed, she would recuff the bottom of her pants, though they barely reached down to the top of her ankles. Occasionally, she'd pull up her red knee socks, scoop up the loose top of each sock with a finger, twist the excess fabric, and tuck it under the rim of the sock to tie it. It was the swiftest set of movements she made.

She pulled over a folding tray table and started scratching dried splotches of spilled coffee off the Formica top. She then smoothed her fine wrinkled hands over the surface. "I . . . I . . ." She seemed to want to say "wash" but finally gave up and uttered, "I scrape it." She continued to seek cleanliness and signs of order in a disintegrating world. She had lost her home, her best friend, and her language—her chief mode of interacting. Yet she still coped and loved the world. She was a favorite of the staff and helped them clean the home. They, in turn, took her with them for rides around the neighborhood.

Eventually, I had to leave. "I'm glad to have had a chance to visit you." Her eyes showed she was trying to understand what I had said. Not until I stood up did she grasp that I was parting. She pulled my arm gently back toward her and kissed me lightly on the cheek. No patient had ever kissed me before. "Last . . ." she uttered. "Last . . . last."

"Last what?" I inquired softly.

She didn't answer.

Stalking the Wild Brain

Once a week, Dr. Spencer held professor rounds. He first visited every patient in the Neuro Intensive Care Unit, and then all the new admissions on the regular neurology ward, walking into each room with a crowd of doctors and medical students in his wake. We followed him through double metal doors inscribed with the name of the unit, below which a second sign bore the handwritten words, "No Flowers Allowed." A medical student in the rear crunched up an empty bag of Lays potato chips as he stuffed the last of the chips into his mouth. An intern read papers on her clipboard as she strolled, checking off chores she had completed.

Dr. William Spencer was a tall man in his late fifties. Though balding, his brown side burns were chiseled precisely, and the lenses of his horn-rimmed glasses always seemed to sparkle, freshly polished. He toted a small briefcase carrying nothing but a tuning fork, a reflex hammer, and a flashlight—the tools of his trade.

The brain is one of three ultimate scientific frontiers, along with the outer rim of the universe and the core of the atom, filled with mesons and quarks. The complex order and encoding of the central nervous system remains to be cracked. To decipher how speech, thought, and personality are mapped in the central gray and white tissue—remains one of the most exciting quests left. Explorers have approached it in a variety of ways. Some researchers have started from the inside out, photographing the tips of neurons and cataloging the chemicals these cells squirt at one another. Other investigators have analyzed the nervous systems of snails, which consist of only a handful of cells. Still others have approached their subject from the outside in, investigating how breakdowns in the nervous system present themselves to the outside world. How do people with broken brains function? What is their behavior? How do they look? This was the method pursued by Dr. Spencer.

"Nothing can substitute for a solid examination of the patient him- or herself," he reminded us. Dr. Spencer believed he could fathom defects in the central nervous system by speaking with and examining the person directly. He was interested in the whole person embodying the brain. He was a naturalist who observed experiments of nature—unplanned accidents and mistakes—and investigated what he could with the naked eye. His approach, though firmly established by great clinicians of the last century, was being threatened in the current age of high-tech brain scans. Reports of Computerized Axial Tomographs, or CAT scanners, Nuclear Magnetic Resonance Scanners, and Positron Emission Tomography Scanners, and pages of computer printouts of lab values now accumulate in the back of patients' charts. "Don't treat lab tests or CAT scans," he urged. "Treat the patient first." He imparted his message principally through teaching rounds. His was the old apprenticeship model. Students observed the master in action.

Neurology cannot always repair the defects it finds. Dr.

Spencer felt challenged by the question of diagnosis and cheered by the accurate answer he often was able to provide where others had failed. He remained excited by the possibility of diagnosing a patient's problem, and undaunted by his often limited power to reverse the damage he discovered.

In the NICU, he led us to the first bed on the right, occupied by Mr. Stuart Beckman.

Mrs. Beckman was standing at her husband's bedside. "Stu, Stu, it's Doris," she was saying in a loud whisper over the noise of the respirator machine hissing and his cardiac monitor squeaking in a high electronic pitch. "How are you doing today?" Mr. Beckman lay motionless.

Mrs. Beckman noticed Dr. Spencer approaching the bedside but turned back to her husband. "Nancy's coming in to visit today," she continued. "I bet you'll be happy to see her. She'll stay for a few days."

Mrs. Beckman, with her two daughters, Nancy and Arlene, kept an around-the-clock vigil by his bedside. They longed for him to be revived. For days at a time one or two of them would camp out on the ward. Unkempt and bedraggled, they resembled a band of gypsies, their few bags of belongings heaped around them as they sat or slept on a wooden bench in the hallway to which they had laid claim. The daughters' quilted shoulder bags would collapse on the floor and spill out wads of moist tissues, a battered box of Kleenex, a bundled-up blouse, a toiletry kit, a thermos, a paperback romance.

Dr. Spencer spoke up. "Would you excuse us?" he asked Mrs. Beckman. "We'd like to examine your husband." Reluctantly, she nodded and retreated before the throng of white uniforms.

I presented Mr. Beckman's history to the group.

He was a sixty-five-year-old married white male, with a long history of hypertension, who three years ago underwent a "cabbage." This is how doctors pronounce the acronym CABG, which stands for Coronary Artery Bypass Graft.

At home, five weeks earlier, Mr. Beckman had been taking two medications, an antihypertensive to lower his blood pressure, and an anticoagulant to "thin" his blood, making it congeal more slowly. Unfortunately, he confused the two little brown bottles of pills. He accidentally swallowed too many anticoagulants and too few antihypertensives. Under the high pressure that ensued, he suffered an intracranial hemorrhage. A vessel in his head burst and the bleeding, once started, didn't stop. On admission, both his blood pressure and his clotting time were dangerously high. A plastic shunt was inserted into his brain to drain the extra fluid into the space around his stomach. He improved, and the day I started on the neurology service, he had been sitting up in bed for the first time.

"Good morning," I said, "I'm your new intern."

He looked up at me and nodded, slightly confused.

"How are you doing?"

"O . . . kay."

I examined him briefly and went on. An hour later, a vessel reburst. His consciousness slipped away and he was "unitized"—shipped across the hall to the Intensive Care Unit, where he had been for the past six days.

There, the parts of his body communicated to me without mediation through him. He couldn't tell me he had shortness of breath, but I counted his respiratory rate when it increased. I inserted an arterial line in his wrist, to gain direct access to his arterial blood supply, and I drew samples. He couldn't complain of dysuria—burning pain on urination—but I saw changes in the color and chemistry of his urine, all of which was trapped and tested. Several times each day, I performed the duties of an integrating mind for his failing body, calculating the homeostatic adjustments in incoming fluid that he was no longer able to perform himself. His thirst mechanism was broken. He couldn't communicate when he was dry. Instead, I estimated out how much water he required by fingering a pocket calculator. If I sped up his infusion rate by ten milliliters an hour, I followed the minute-to-minute reactions of his blood pressure and pulse. He was a crucible in which I tinkered. Every orifice of his body was crammed with tubes through which various fluids flowed in and out. Every limb was punctured. Urine catheter, NG tube, IV tubes, chest tube, trach tube, rectal tube. His body lay inert, sapped. Three times a day, the ICU nurse, Donna, would turn him on one side or the other to avoid bedsores.

The morning of professor rounds, as soon as Mrs. Beckman left the room, Dr. Spencer bent forward toward Mr. Beckman's face. "Stuu, Stuuuu," he coaxed. The skin didn't flicker. Spencer stood up, then bent down again, nearing the patient. "Mr. Beckman, are you with us?" There was no response. He clapped his hands loudly by the patient's ear, then slapped his hand on the bed. There was no sign of life. Spencer lifted one of the patient's fluid-swollen fingers and pressed the edge of a pen against the fingernail. The limp hand twitched. "What do you conclude?" Spencer asked me.

"He responds to pain."

"Don't be vague in your language. Do not say that he responds to pain. Say that he withdraws to pain. The organism's response to pain is not conscious.

"What's his fluid status?" Dr. Spencer went on.

"His pulse is elevated but he's becoming edematous."

"Are we giving him too much or too little fluid?" Either was plausible. "Do we know his filling pressure?"

I had anticipated this question. A few hours earlier that morning, I had obtained the answer. To know whether the

amount of fluid being pumped into him was appropriate, I had
to measure the pressure in his heart by inserting into that organ
a Swan-Ganz catheter. To perform this task, I had dressed in
a special sterile blue gown and white gloves. Donna had assisted me, unfolding a sterile blue cloth and stretching it over
him like a flag draped over a military corpse. I had uncoiled
the bright yellow plastic catheter. Purple markings were ticked
off on it which would measure the distance traveled toward his
heart.

On top of Mr. Beckman's chest, I had laid out the "swan,"
as it's called—the catheter with four long tails splayed out like
the tentacles of a squid, each available for pumping in a different kind of fluid or medication. With Donna rigorously pre-
serving a sterile field around me, I blew air in from a syringe,
making the balloon on the tip of the catheter bulge and become
visible. When the plunger sucked the air back out, the balloon
disappeared. I lanced the rubbery skin of his neck with a
needle until blood flowed out, demonstrating that it had tapped
his vein. I slipped a thin guide wire through the bore and
removed the needle. The wire stuck out of his neck, and over
it I threaded a plastic sheath, at the external tip of which was
positioned a white cone through which I then removed the wire
and inserted the "swan." On the oscilloscope above his head,
the wave forms told me when I reached his throbbing ventricle.
The "swanning," as this process is called, proceeded without
complications. The barometer housed in the tip measured Mr.
Beckman's cardiac functioning and how much fluid he could
tolerate. The peaks of the oscilloscope wave rose and fell, and
indicated that more fluid was needed.

When Dr. Spencer asked me about the patient's fluid status
on rounds, I was able to answer by reporting the filling pressure.

"Have you increased the IV rate as a result?" he asked.

"Yes, sir. I did."

"How long has this patient been comatose?" he asked.

"One week. Since he came into the unit."

"His prognosis is poor," Spencer mused. "Is he DNR?"

"No." Everything possible was still being done to keep Mr. Beckman viable.

Dr. Spencer furrowed his brow. "Why are we keeping this lifeless collection of organs alive?" he whispered. I had wondered that myself as well. But Dr. Spencer carried more authority than I did to address this question.

"Dr. Barnes is the attending," I said.

"I'll have to speak with him."

"I think we need an ethics consult, stat," I suggested to another intern standing beside me.

"Beckman belongs in a vegetable patch," he retorted.

"What do you mean?"

"His diagnosis is Rule Out Vegetable."

Patient's diagnoses are often presented as "ruling out" a disease. It means that a certain condition is suspected, but that further diagnostic tests are required before proving or disproving the hypothesis. When a patient is admitted to the hospital with chest pain, for example, the intern needs to demonstrate whether he's having a heart attack or just aching ribs. The patient is labeled a "ROMI," an acronym for "Rule Out Myocardial Infarction."

Professor Spencer started to leave the bed, but halted abruptly and turned as a thought seized him. "I was once called to see a patient to rule out life." This term was new to me.

Dr. Spencer explained. "The patient had a pacemaker that beat his heart and was hooked up to a respirator machine that did his breathing. He had perpetual paralysis secondary to Guillain-Barré syndrome. His neurological damage was extensive, and everyone thought he was dead. I was called to confirm this, but I thought I noticed a subtle change in the expression of his eyes. I came by with a lantern and a magnifying glass, held the lens up to the patient's eye, and leaned over him. The lights in the room were shut off and I raised the lantern up, flooding his face with light. Other doctors and nurses crowded around me. Through my lens, I saw the pupils were constricting by half a millimeter in response to the light. 'He's alive,' I said. The room lights were flicked back on." The verdict had been pronounced.

Dr. Spencer marched over to the second bed in the ICU. Mrs. Kennon had locked-in syndrome. Her whole body was paralyzed except for her eyelids and the muscles that moved her eyes. The two eye movements she could make, up and down, were the only two voluntary movements her whole body performed, besides blinking, the only two gestures that told us that she was alert and could hear and think and feel.

"Can you see me?" he asked. "Look up if you can." She did. I assumed therefore that she was not blind. But Dr. Spencer suspected she might be vainly lying.

"Look down," he commanded her. She did. Disconnecting the endotracheal tube that tunneled through the cartilage of her neck into her throat, the professor ordered her, "Hold your breath." She continued to take determined gasps. "Take a deep breath." Again, there was no change.

"Frontal eye fields," Spencer announced, throwing his keys up in the air and catching them in his hand, his eyes traveling up and down, following the trajectory of the flying glint of metal. "Occipital eye fields," he said, throwing the keys at me unexpectedly, everyone's gaze moving sideways to follow them. I was startled but caught them. "The ability to move your eyes without moving your head is an enormous evolutionary advantage. It's often the first thing to go in Huntington's chorea and several other neurological diseases."

Huntington's chorea is a disease marked by choreoathetoid

movements (from the Greek for "dancing without position")—
uncontrollable, twisting arm motions. The illness runs in families and lacks a cure. Woody Guthrie witnessed this disease
slowly grip his body. His son, Arlo, knows his chances of
contracting it. This genetic disease arrived in the New World
on the *Mayflower* and has been passed on in old American
families ever since. In the nineteenth century, sailors to the
South Pacific visiting various islands frolicked on hot tropical
nights beneath the palms, and left their seed, by way of which
the disease continues to sprout on the islands centuries later.
The disease doesn't manifest its cruel symptoms until the fifth
or sixth decade, after having already been sown in the genes
of one or two further generations.

Professor Spencer continued to discuss Mrs. Kennon's case
in front of her. "She's obviously a bright woman," he said at one
point, peering down at her. Her eyes sank away from us briefly.
"None of us would ever want to have a tube in our mouth and be
unable to speak." She looked down again. It was the only set of
gestures she could make. Dr. Spencer continued to analyze her
before the pack of doctors and students, citing her as a sample
of impaired neurological hardware, a malfunctioning computer.
My eyes glanced down with hers.

Sitting up in the next bed was Mrs. Roberta Swanson. A
rare ICU patient, she was alert. She had been admitted to the
hospital a few days earlier with a brain tumor and had been
sent to the operating room. Unfortunately, the "gumba," as a
tumor is called, turned out to be too big and too firmly embedded in the rest of her brain to be fully excised. The surgeon,
Dr. Barnes, had removed only a small portion of it to send as
a biopsy rather than take out the whole mass as he had planned.
The cancer would stay in her skull and grow at its own—one
hoped slow—pace.

Following this procedure yesterday, she was sent to the ICU, as had been planned beforehand when it had been anticipated that she would be recovering from major surgery. She awoke there this morning as she had expected, ignorant of the change in tactics. She had quietly observed Donna washing Mr. Beckman and had listened to Dr. Spencer discourse on the other patients.

"Good day, madam," Dr. Spencer greeted her, nodding.

"Hello. Can I read?" she asked me. *The New York Times* was already propped up on her lap.

"Yes, of course," I answered, glancing toward Dr. Spencer. "How are you doing?"

"Great," she said with a big smile.

"Really?"

"I'm so lucky," she said, putting the paper down by her side.

"Why is that?"

"Because I went through an operation which everyone said was going to be horribly difficult and traumatic, and I'm still alive and feel fine." I realized the gravity of her delusion. What could I say? Should I further the deception?

"Did Dr. Barnes come by yet?"

"No, I haven't seen him since before the operation." It was his job to inform her what he had and hadn't accomplished. Maybe he had come by when she was still lethargic from the anesthesia. Perhaps the burden delayed him. I wasn't about to scoop him in transmitting the news.

"Aren't I lucky?" she repeated innocently, as I mulled over these thoughts.

"Yes," I said and sighed, "I think you are."

"Can you answer a question?" she asked, unaware of my hesitation. "How long do I have to stay in here?"

Machines flickered, buzzed, rang, purred, hummed, beeped, and clicked all around her.

"I'm not sure. We'll have to check with Dr. Barnes."

"Hopefully, not long at all," Dr. Spencer added. This environment can discombobulate patients, depriving them of customary sensory stimuli and flooding them with others—fluorescent lights, and nurses puttering twenty-four hours to a cacophony of machines. Patients on high doses of painkillers, sleeping pills, and anti-anxiety medications may become confused. Some even develop delusional beliefs that they are somewhere else, or that their mother is standing in the hallway, though she might have been dead for years.

When we were out of earshot, Dr. Spencer turned to us. "Make sure you talk to Dr. Barnes about her this morning. I want her out of here. She shouldn't be occupying a unit bed. It may hurt her more than help her."

Since Dr. Spencer had handed down his opinion, she would probably be discharged that afternoon directly from the ICU to her home.

Dr. Spencer sped onto the regular ward, his head lowered, sunk in thought. We followed him to see Stacey Neal, who had been admitted the night before. I presented her case in the hallway. By this point in the year, I had learned how to encapsulate a patient's story concisely. She was a twenty-one-year-old college junior at Sarah Lawrence, scheduled to start her next semester in a few days, who complained of odd headaches and pains in the middle of her back. Her physical exam was normal. But when tested for muscle strength, she had "given way." That is, when I requested she hold her hands up and not let me push her away, she at first resisted, but then dropped one arm limply to her flank. Stacey had probably wagered that this was a sure sign of neurological disease. But it only indicated that she had cheated on the exam. Genuine muscle weakness is constant. She would have been unable to oppose my force at all.

"How are you doing this morning, Miss Neal?" I asked her as we crowded around her bed.

"I had a headache last night at the place where I said my hair hurt." Hair rarely hurts. I asked her to hold her hands out in the air in front of her while closing her eyes, another exam used to detect brain disease. I watched to see whether one or both arms drifted through the air instead of remaining stationary. It's an old test, and Miss Neal, who had managed to have herself admitted to the hospital seven other times in the past two years, was no doubt familiar with it. She shut her eyes, and started bouncing her arms in the air. Her movements were not at all those of a patient with neurological damage. My colleagues and I rolled our eyes at each other, and spilled out of her room into the hallway.

"Have you ever heard of the ankle bracelet sign?" Spencer asked me. A gold-plated bracelet inscribed with her name in script graced her ankle.

"No, what is it?"

"Fifty percent of patients who wear them fake their symptoms."

"Is that true?"

"A study was actually once done on this."

Professor Spencer leaned forward. "Most back pain is in the cervical or lumbar portions of the vertebral column and not in the thoracic region, where she's complaining of it. That is, most back pain is a pain in the neck or a pain in the ass. That's why those expressions are common in our speech. It's usually muscle pain, emotionally related, with or without some nerve root disease. But pain in the middle of the back is unusual." The motives for Miss Neal's deceit didn't intrigue him.

"Who's the next patient?" he asked. We visited Victor Sandoz, a twenty-seven-year-old Hispanic male with a very slow-growing brain tumor. He was mildly mentally retarded and without growth hormone. He looked ten years old. His mother blamed his small size on the fact that she had fallen once during the pregnancy. Patients and their families frequently cite an event—an accident, or even a divorce—as the precipitating cause of an illness. If the origin of an illness is understood, they believe a cure might be as well. But Mrs. Sandoz's fall was unrelated to his defect.

During the day, he attended a special training program, building model airplanes in a woodworking shop. He had no complaints now except occasional headaches.

"Do you know where you are?" the professor asked him.

"No." On his night stand sat a small wooden propeller plane.

"No idea?"

"They tell me I'm in the hospital." He picked up the plane. "Vrum, Vrumm, Vrummm," he hummed as he guided the aircraft through the air in front of him before landing it beside the pillow on his bed.

"Yes, it's hard to believe but it's true."

We gathered back out in the hallway. Spencer looked at all of us and said, "Should we give him growth hormones, or operate?" The patient was already slated for the operating room for the next morning. "What would his life be like if we went into his head? Can we make him a happier human being?" He looked out a nearby window. A morning mist shifted through the city, erasing whole portions of buildings. Victor was happy but neurologically impaired, a simpleton. Brain surgery might make him more intelligent and prolong his life, or it might be traumatic and fail, rendering him far more neurologically damaged than he now was. Slicing with a knife through a brain could be catastrophic—even with the most skillful hand pushing the scalpel. Victor was content without the procedure, innocent of his defect.

Spencer replied to his own question. "Maybe we can make him happier," he said. "Maybe." But Dr. Spencer's reflections wouldn't influence the established plans.

We walked to the foot of the bed next door. Mrs. Shabaz Nimori was a forty-year-old Iranian woman whose spinal cord had been transected to remove a tumor that had grown there, leaving her quadriplegic, paralyzed below her neck. Since she was unable to breathe, a tracheotomy had been performed, and she had been hooked up ever since via plastic tubing to a machine with twenty black dials on it that breathed for her through the surgically made hole in her throat. Unable to speak, she could only whisper and pant. Her husband, a short timorous Iranian man, had visited her the previous night and had spoon-fed her Persian food. Partially masticated lamb and potatoes conglomerated in the corner of her mouth and dribbled down her chin.

"Any problems today?" I asked.

She blinked her eyes twice, a prearranged sign for "yes." One blink meant "no."

"What's the matter?"

"Ssssechinng," she mumbled faintly.

"Suctioning?" I guessed she was referring to the process by which nurses cleaned out her mucus-laden tube.

"Saachonning." She mouthed the sounds.

"Oxygen?" I said, as if playing a guessing game.

"Pachishoi."

"Poisongel?" I invented a word that seemed closest to her sounds. She remained calm throughout this interchange, which was vital to her despite its exhausting absurdity to me.

"Sasishoning."

"Positioning?" I tried, referring to the tube or other parts of her paralyzed body.

She blinked her eyes firmly twice. I readjusted the position of the tubing at her throat.

Dr. Spencer turned to the group. "What are you doing with her?"

"She spiked again last night," I informed him.

The night before, she had been febrile. I had suspected a pneumonia, and had talked with my resident about her.

"X-ray, culture, and blood gas her," he had advised. I sent off sputum, blood, and urine cultures and a sample of arterial blood. Also, a portable X-ray machine was brought to her bedside since she couldn't leave her room. A nurse and I had lifted her up, hauling her torso forward. The X-ray film sealed in a thick case was wedged between her injured spine and her pillows. We eased her paralyzed body back down. The radiology technician brought up his machine and aimed the head of his contraption at her chest. The metal monster had a long multi-jointed neck, enabling it to bend in any direction. A small head took the pictures and a heavy body supported on motorized wheels contained a control panel. The technician slipped on a leaded smock. "X-ray!" he shouted. Passersby in the hall scattered. No one is ever sure how far to stand from the machine, how far to escape, how much to be inconvenienced. Did the rays penetrate through doors? Windows? Walls? Was the doorway safe, the opposite wall or down the hall? With a high-pitched electronic hum, the photo was snapped. The film demonstrated an infection and I started triple antibiotics—amp, clinda, and gent. These three antibiotics— ampicillin, clindamycin, and gentamycin—would cover organisms she might be harboring. Infection, though, was a secondary problem.

"Has she changed neurologically at all in the past few weeks?" Spencer asked me.

"She hasn't. Could anything help her?"

Spencer shook his head. "There's nothing else to do. The best we can hope for is to place her somewhere good."

In the last room on the hall sat Mrs. Hathaway, an eighty-year-old biologist who had been in good health until yesterday, when she abruptly became confused. She probably had had a stroke. She had come to the Emergency Room, where the doctor who saw her wrote in his note that she was "loquacious and euphoric." I had started her on medicine to thin her blood.

"Push out your cheeks," Dr. Spencer instructed her now. In her pink silk bathrobe, bedecked with pearls and diamond earrings, she distorted her face. "Show us your teeth," Dr. Spencer demanded. She approximated a smile.

"Can you write a sentence for us? How about: 'Today is Tuesday'?" She tried but got stuck on the third or fourth letter. She stopped and looked up at us.

"Oh, look, it's really nice of you to come around," she said, putting the pen down, "but I have to go now. Would you be so kind as to go summon me a cab?"

"But, Mrs. Hathaway, you'll be staying here at the hospital tonight," I told her.

"Oh, look, that's awfully nice of you to offer and to spend all this time with me, but if you could just get me a cab . . ."

"Can you repeat after me: 'No ifs, ands, or buts'?" Dr. Spencer interrupted. This was a standard line used to test if a patient's motor speech is broken.

"No ifs . . . You've all been very kind, you really have been."

"How about: 'Methodist Episcopal'?"

"Metho . . ."

Her damaged brain neglected the left side of her visual field, and as we encircled her, she suddenly remembered the professor who had entered with us and was now standing at the left side of her bed. "Where did that older gentleman go?" Mrs. Hathaway suddenly inquired, perplexed. We said nothing but exchanged glances among ourselves. Sensing our awkwardness, Mrs. Hathaway turned her head from one side to the other and finally spotted him. "Oh, there he is," she said jocosely as if nothing had happened, not the least concerned about her new deficit. Nonchalance is a common symptom of a recent stroke.

Dr. Spencer paused in the hallway, his briefcase at his side. Rounds were over. "We all think we see everything. But I am aware at all times that I only see through a porthole, and am surrounded by a white wall. Our fields of vision are always confined."

IV. Deviations

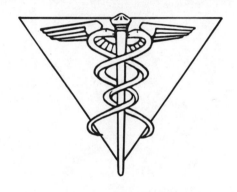

Good Hands

"Take as much blood as you need," Mrs. Sarah Greer encouraged me. She had just arrived on the obstetrics and gynecology ward, and I was drawing blood for routine preoperative tests. She looked too healthy to be in the hospital.

Sarah dreamed of having children. She and her husband had tried without success. She was now thirty-eight; her fortieth birthday was their deadline. Her two sisters both had kids. Her mother had delivered all three of them by the time she was Sarah's age.

Two years earlier, the Greers had visited Dr. Conrad and had undergone a series of tests. He'd concluded that the problem was blockage of her Fallopian tubes. The solution was surgical, excising ova, or eggs, from her ovaries for *in vitro* fertilization, or IVF, that is, fertilization in a test tube outside her body.

"Do you think the procedure will work?" she asked me.

"It might. Dr. Conrad has an impressive rate of success comparatively, but there's no guarantee."

"We've been through a lot."

"You're in good hands."

Dr. Conrad scheduled her operation for 7:00 A.M. That morning, I walked into the locker room and changed into freshly washed blue surgical robes. The uniform was faded, washed after each operation it had witnessed. I covered my head with a paper cap and pulled paper covers with elastic rims over my running shoes. I softly padded down the hall. Janitors hauling carts of supplies were identically clad.

"They're still cleaning up from the last operation," Dr. Conrad told me when I arrived. "We'll be backed up for an hour." He paced the antechamber in front of the operating room, informing new arrivals of the delay and pressing the janitors who were cleaning up to hurry. Every few seconds he shot an angry, impatient glance at them from behind his spectacles. In his mid-fifties, he had helped pioneer these surgical techniques. He rarely had time to spare.

I wandered out to the staff lounge. Surgeons had their own private retreat. In the staff lounge, scrub nurses, technicians, and medical students, some of them asleep, sat in plastic chairs around a central table that supported an urn of drab coffee, a box of graham crackers, and jars of generic peanut butter with wooden tongue depressors jammed into them. Yesterday's newspaper lay on the Formica top, the ink blurred where coffee had spilled. These snacks didn't constitute a normal breakfast, but they were what we all ate.

When the operating time approached, I went into the intermediary scrub room, where, along one wall, there was a long troughlike metal sink equipped with pedals that turned on hot and cold water. I removed three sponges, each wrapped separately in a silver package, to sterilize myself. Imbedded in each was a thin plastic wedge to scrape out any grime beneath my fingernails. With each sponge, I lathered the suds from my fingertips to my elbows. Three times I soaped and rinsed. I walked into the OR immaculate.

Mrs. Greer lay on the table. Dr. Conrad coated her groin and her belly with three washes of iodine antiseptic soap. He and I spread out sterile blue and gray cloth drapes with holes cut in them, which we positioned over her inguinal and umbilical areas. "I'm going to be giving you some nice drugs, here," Dr. Gaittens, the anesthesiologist, was saying. "You'll be dropping off to sleep in no time. You won't feel a thing." Her eyes looked up at him. She smiled and her eyes shut. "You can't get drugs like this anywhere else, so enjoy the ride." He smiled underneath his mask.

"Looks like she's gone," he said.

"That seemed fast," I commented, standing near him.

He pumped a rubber oxygen bag with his hand. "Anesthesia is like flying," he said as he quickly replaced the bag with a ventilation mask connected to an oxygen tank. "The dangerous parts are takeoff and landing. The rest is easy." He seated himself on a stool by her head, behind a fence of glass cylinders with bubbles buoyed between calibrations, measuring gas pressures.

"What do we have scheduled after this?" Conrad asked the nurse.

"A 'D and C,' " meaning a dilation and curettage.

"Let me have a scalpel," he said. He made a small incision on Mrs. Greer's abdomen just below her navel, drawing a thin bright red line. He etched the line a second time, more deeply, and blood welled up into the fissure. His scalpel penetrated farther, through other layers of skin and tissue. He then inserted a laparoscope—a long tube with an eyepiece at one end, a flexible fiberoptic telescope that gave him visual access to her ovaries. He made another incision in her groin and inserted a fine suction needle, with which he extracted an egg. He carried the specimen swiftly to his microscope, sterilely set up against the wall. Into the clear fluid of a shallow circular glass dish—a petri dish—he dropped his find.

"Nurse, hand me a probe." His eyes didn't lift from his microscope lens, where he was hunched, examining his prize. He eased the fragile egg along with the tip of his metal instrument.

"Can I take a peek?" I asked.

"Just a minute," he said, still studying it. "All right, go ahead," he finally said, backing off abruptly.

I had never seen even a photo of a human egg before. I had admired color photographs of fetuses in *Life* magazine, floating in their amniotic balloons like space capsules. Peering through the microscope, I saw a glistening egg on a background of clear white space. The bright yellow orb shone like a small sun, its round edge surrounded by a reflecting white halo of pearl jello. This thin milky veil spread around the yolk like an egg white. The egg looked like one from a chicken, spilled from its shell onto a griddle. Nothing about it appeared related to human life.

My high school biology teacher had once proudly displayed to the class his son's umbilical cord and amniotic sac, which he had preserved. It would be disturbing to have a father show this beige, brown, yellow, and black jellyfish-like mass to his own son, even at an age when he might understand it, and say, "This was once attached to you." An egg and a person were as difficult to reconcile, as radically disconnected. But I now saw a clear similarity between animals and man. A few genes more or less inside the yolk make all the difference.

This ovum appeared special, however, magnified in the microscope's eyepiece and covering the entire eye field. It possessed the aura of a beehive seen through a plate of glass, observed carrying out a complex encoded order. This sealed envelope contained all the vital information that would get handed down genetically, beyond language. It recorded someone's fate. Going to medical school seemed worthwhile just to view this extraordinary sight.

I yielded the scope back to Dr. Conrad, whose trained eye would judge whether this cell was viable enough to be fertilized, fit enough to become a person. I watched his face to divine his impression.

"How do you tell?" I asked.

"By looking at it, whether it seems like it'll make it or not."

"What do you look for exactly?"

"For example, whether it's lopsided or whole."

While he examined his egg, the surgical nurse was busy replenishing her tray of hooks, scalpels, forceps, and pincers, arranged in size order on a steel gray cloth. She laid out handfuls of probes with tips curved like fingers used for burrowing beneath layers of muscle, ready for Dr. Conrad if he decided to probe further.

Dr. Conrad had been one of the pioneers in this technique of technological sex. The procedure was performed very naturally and matter-of-factly, as if it were the most common thing in the world. Little was explained. The nurses and anesthesiologist went about their assigned tasks as if it were a routine hernia operation. Where was the ritual or celebration appropriate to this feat?

"No good!" he barked at last. "We need more eggs." He hurried toward the patient, extracted another, and examined it.

"Great . . . it looks fantastic!" he suddenly yelled, his hands fluttering up into the air. "We did it!" I wanted to inspect the winning sample. But to me it would probably look similar to the one he had rejected, which had seemed beautifully proportioned to me.

Dr. Conrad gathered an extra two eggs, in case the one he liked didn't fertilize, and the operation ended. Mrs. Greer's incision was closed.

The eggs were fertilized in a test tube, and two days later implanted in Mrs. Greer's uterus. She stayed in the hospital another two days. When I last saw her, she was sitting on the edge of her bed, waiting for her husband to arrive and take her home. She smiled politely at me but seemed tentative and timid. The overall success rate of *in vitro* fertilization was not high.

I never saw her again, but many months later I learned from Dr. Conrad that Mrs. Greer had given birth to a son.

Cyclops

O ne afternoon, I took a shortcut from the ward to one of the labs. I accidentally stumbled through an anatomy corridor the likes of which I hadn't seen since my first year of medical school four years earlier. Tall wooden display cases from the last century lined the walls. In these glass cabinets, shelves displayed abnormal fetuses. In gallon-sized jars filled with formaldehyde, these creatures, which had spontaneously aborted, hung suspended in the greenish tint of their under-water worlds. These pink leathery beings had arrested at various points in their gestation—at 5 weeks, 10 weeks, 20 weeks, 25—their physical features slowly becoming recognizable as human. Their snouts had become noses, their appendages hands with fingers rather than hoofs or claws. But errors were made. One fetus had sprouted two heads, another had grown a large pedicle as a single leg. Nature had weeded out these sprigs, deeming them unfit.

One of these rejects was a cyclops. Its eye opened from beneath wide lids on its forehead, where two eyes would ordinarily be. The creature gazed out, its wrinkled fingers extended, palms flat against the jar. Its forehead and single eye pressed against the glass, staring blankly through the formaldehyde.

Cyclopes exist. Perhaps one of these innocent and pathetic creatures was born (or aborted) in ancient Greece and, thanks to the power of its allegoric implications, became the stuff of legend. Its neighbor in the showcase, a one-legger, was curious but had fewer metaphorical possibilities. In a society that places primacy on sight, one-eyed vision has a lot of potential. Did it see only half as much, or was it only half as smart? Did the Greeks realize that it was the presence of two eyes that enabled human beings to see three-dimensionally? Animals with eyes facing outward from the sides of their heads see different, often barely overlapping, scenes in the environment. Those scenes are flat. Evolution slowly shifted the eyes closer together and nearer to the front of the head. Man is he who, more than any other animal, sees in 3-D. All animals, from fish on up, have two eyes. Was a creature with only one eye not only nonhuman but nonanimal as well? Was it for this reason that the poor cyclops was said to be a monster, neither beast nor man?

The next jar on the shelf displayed spina bifida, a spinal cord that never fused during the development of the fetus. The spinal canal opened to the outside, exposing the brain directly to the environment. The brain experienced the world without mediation. Temperature would not have to be reported via thermal receptors in the skin passing their information back to the brain neuron by neuron. The brain wouldn't learn of the temperature fourth-, fifth-, or one thousandth-handed. I know I am cold when my skin tells my brain it's cold, goosefleshed, and shivering. In spina bifida, the unclothed brain itself would become chilled. Unfortunately, the organism wouldn't survive.

The womb was the scene of the first step in the evolutionary process of selection. Not all types of fetuses survive. This anatomy museum noted the ones that had failed. Students scurrying through this back corridor rarely glanced at the small index cards of dense type bearing the smack of a manual typewriter. The fetuses drifted in their preserver fluid, suspended in time. They lived only weeks. They are preserved forever.

The doors beside these glass cases led into the Gross Anatomy suites. I assumed that the name of this academic discipline referred to the study of the entire human body at a macroscopic level, and that the other connotation of the term "gross" was unintentional. In these rooms, corpses lay on six-foot-long tables for use in anatomical dissections. These bodies concealed hearts that had beat over decades rather than weeks, yet the corpses were cut up each semester, their amputated parts pitched into wastebaskets till all that remained was flesh clinging to bones, reminiscent of a roasted turkey the day after Thanksgiving.

Medicine is particularly interested in understanding the losers. Its chief concern is, after all, things going wrong with the functioning of a biological organism. No other field is more focused on studying errors. Yet no other field so avoids examining its own mistakes or even admitting that it makes them. Lawyers would never imagine that they were gods. Doctors presume it daily.

We think of deviancy in sociological terms—criminals, drug addicts, and their ilk. But these glass jars reminded us of nature's undesirables. Their arms spread against the glass, they looked as if they sought to escape the confines of their cylindrical prisons, to interact with us, to enter the mainstream, to be part of us and our definition of ourselves.

Dr. Donald Toller, who had collected these specimens, was raised in rural Georgia. Each day in class, he played a videotape of the dissection that students were to perform and announced over the intercom with a Southern drawl, "Okay, everybody, here's the tape."

At one point, probably back in the last century, anatomy had been a cornerstone of medical education, a respectable academic discipline. But clinical medicine changed. Advanced research in other fields discovered new enzymes, drugs, hormones, and antibodies, uncovering how cells divide, and how cancer sparks and grows. Technology jetted on, leaving him and his field behind. Not much new was being discovered about gross anatomy anymore. The body remained unchanged. Techniques of dissecting a cadaver hadn't advanced much either, not since the Renaissance. The scalpel remained the cutting edge.

Though once the Department of Anatomy had been a full academic department, it had since been demoted in status to being a subsection of the Department of Surgery.

Dr. Toller studied the evolution of man from apes. I had never met as confirmed and committed an evolutionist who viewed human beings first and foremost as having descended from primates. He saw the hands and feet of human beings as similar to those of apes. The same areas of the brain that make chimps get antsy made men feel anxious as well. Men got into wars in part because of inherited neuronal pathways. Dr. Toller talked about the mating patterns of chimps, and noted those of medical students, too.

He wondered what our ancestors, the Neanderthals, were like. Though they probably breeded like us, they couldn't have talked much, he would say. Only after the vocal tract evolved further was it able to produce more sounds, and only then make a language with words. He argued that language was invented not when the human brain attained the capacity to handle a symbolic universe, but only after the muscles and cartilage of the throat had toughened and expanded. Man needed more muscle, not more brain, to be able to develop language.

Dr. Toller was a passionate teacher.

He preserved a fresh rawness and enthusiasm as he wandered from cadaver to cadaver. "Have you found the spleen yet?" he asked me one day.

"No. I tried but couldn't locate it." I had fished with my hand gently along the inside of the cadaver's ribs down the left side. Cold slippery organs had swallowed my fingers. I had concluded that the spleen was absent.

"Here. Let me do it," Dr. Toller said.

He plunged his arm in up to his elbow, cast about, and rose back to the surface with the rounded organ in his hand. It had been lodged farther back than I had ventured.

He loved knowing that students were learning, fingering the slipperiness of human fat, tearing, poking, and palming flesh. Soon, the pages of my textbook felt oily, smeared with the grease of various organs, and splattered with specks that had been flicked up into the air during particularly strenuous sessions of cutting and sawing.

Anatomy was the first class to be taken when one arrived in medical school. One had to master the dead before handling the living. One of the members of my four-person dissection group was Katherine, a petite woman with short blond hair. She hailed from Virginia, a descendant of an old Virginia family, and had attended a Southern women's college. Since her sophomore year, her father had been ill with cancer. Her mother had died when she was eight. I was never sure whether Katherine was motivated to come to medical school as a result of these experiences. In any case, early on she found herself hacking open corpses and allowing the heavy smell of formaldehyde to permeate her Anne Klein clothes. Although the class generally wore disposable flesh-colored rubber gloves

188 / A Year-long Night

during dissections, Katherine had managed to find the equivalent glove in pink. Delicacy was somehow preserved.

The corpse was kept covered, except for the one portion being explored. When I opened the abdomen, I kept the remainder—the chest, head, limbs, and groin—hidden beneath sheets. When I cracked open the ribs and delved into the chest, the head and everything below the waist were concealed. As the semester wore on, these distinctions became increasingly difficult to maintain. Flaps of skin became more numerous, the corpse more revealed, less remaining unsullied. Katherine sought to preserve the decorum. Most other anatomy groups dumped the sheet haphazardly onto a corner of the leftover corpse. But Katherine neatly pulled the large greenish black rubber sheet completely over the body each day with the firm decisiveness of one who is upholding a moral order.

Toward the end of the term, the week arrived when we would dissect genitalia. We watched a five-minute summary of the procedure we were to perform—two-and-a-half minutes of dissecting a female, and two-and-a-half minutes of doing the equivalent to a male. Male organs were to be sliced through in two dimensions, female genitalia were to be split, parting the two sides. It was the most troubling dissection yet. "I want everyone doing this dissection," Dr. Toller said.

"How crude he is!" Katherine protested when the videotape came to an end. She held back at first as the dissection began, turning her head away with an air of disgust, but unable to resist peering over at us to see what we three others were doing. "I'll hand you the instruments," she declared.

After a day or two, it was clear that all the rest of the class were busied in their work. "I'll read the instructions for the procedure to you," she said. But there wasn't much to read.

Finally, Katherine reluctantly joined in. She resigned herself to holding up a flap of skin here and there, averting her face.

But it wasn't as repulsive as she had feared. She began to glance over her shoulder, and she became interested. She turned to watch, and then joined in the dissection. "Here, I'll do that, Bob," she said about the next step in the cutting. Soon, she was asking me to hand her the instruments. Her curiosity awoke.

Our corpse was male. I didn't know if she had ever had this much exposure to flesh of the opposite sex. But here was a "safe" environment in which to explore it.

Toward the end of our dissection, Dr. Toller made an announcement: "Since all of you have either a male or a female corpse, you all should visit neighboring groups working on a cadaver of the opposite sex." The tables of corpses lay parallel, lined up down the center of the long room like beds in an old-fashioned hospital ward. The four women at the next table had a female corpse. We visited them and they gave us a tour of their work. We in turn gave them a description of our findings. Each group visited another team's table.

Katherine became fascinated. Soon she was visiting still other groups, approaching all the teams working on male cadavers and receiving the standard tour. She became a class expert on variations between the cadavers. It was the most interaction she had had thus far with some students in the class as she approached them and inspected their work.

Dr. Toller had continued to have an important lesson to teach.

Baby Girl Cooke

From the sealed windows in the Newborn Medical Special Care Unit, I watched the sun beat a soft glow onto the concrete hospital buildings. A sudden ring startled me. The phone labeled "Hot Line" was summoning pediatricians to the delivery room.

Grabbing a tool kit filled with equipment needed in "high risk" deliveries, I rushed down the hall. The supply box of syringes, suction tubes, drugs, and oxygen masks clunked along at my side.

I walked into the delivery room, which was dimly lit, with the curtains pulled shut. Henry Cooke held his wife, Pamela, one hand embracing her bent knee, the other hand entwined with hers. She had been infected during her pregnancy with the parasite *Toxoplasma gondii*. The Cookes had been told that their first child might emerge into the world deformed, perhaps already dead. Amniocentesis and ultrasound had failed to determine this with any certainty. We'd have to wait to see the infant in the flesh.

Toxoplasmosis is everywhere. It spreads through cysts that lie in soil or through the feces of birds and small mammals, including cats. If a woman becomes infected during pregnancy, her fetus, whose immune system develops slowly, is unable to fend off the invader and can be severely damaged.

The obstetrician, Dr. Janet Grover, explored Mrs. Cooke's cervix with gloved fingers. "The baby's head is wide," she announced. Atop Mrs. Cooke's swollen belly she placed an electronic stethoscope which she plugged into an oscilloscope. Across a lit green screen, lights blinked and bounced, tracing the pulsations of a tiny heart within the womb. A digital counter flashed the heart rate, and red lights marked the beat. Everyone but Mrs. Cooke watched the screen. In those electronic bleeps I sensed the immediacy of a human inching toward us. But those delicate vibrations could be stifled in the birth canal. The baby could emerge dead or deformed.

Mrs. Cooke's contractions became more frequent; her cervix widened. A fuzzy scalp appeared. Two ears flopped free. "Stop pushing," Dr. Grover instructed her. "Breathe out slowly . . . relax." The head emerged, and then shoulders and trunk slid out effortlessly. Chubby legs kicked air for the first time. Forceps clamped and scissors sliced the twisted cord.

The child breathed, though haltingly. It stirred, then wailed as Dr. Grover wiped it off and fumbled with it.

"What is it?" Mrs. Cooke begged, straining to glimpse the scene between her knees.

"It's a girl," Dr. Grover announced. Robed, hooded, and masked, she held the child up to its mother. The infant's left arm was twisted and shrunken, however, and its face lopsided. No one mentioned the obvious and frightening defects.

"Oh, honey," Mrs. Cooke exclaimed to her husband, seeing her first child before her, distorted but crying. "It's a girl!" Mr. Cooke stared, dazed at the deformed infant. "Did you hear that?" she repeated, unaware of his reaction. "We have a baby girl."

No one said "It's a baby," "It's injured," or "It's alive."

"The baby might have some problems," someone said cautiously to Mrs. Cooke. "We'll have to take her to the Special Care nursery to be watched."

"It's a girl, honey. We've had a girl!" Mrs. Cooke cried again, ignoring the rest of what had been said.

Mutely, her husband patted her shoulder.

I wrapped the baby in a white towel and carried her down the hall to the Neonatal ICU. The child now had a medical problem, requiring the care of pediatricians, not the obstetrician who had followed Mrs. Cooke in her pregnancy and delivery. In the Newborn Special Care Unit, I lifted the Lucite lid of an empty isolation box and placed her inside. The roof snapped shut. On the front of this "basin," as it's called, two round portholes permitted passage of a nurse or doctor's aseptically gloved hands to provide care to the infant. Oxygen and heat were pumped in. Soon, with eyes shut, the baby groped with her legs and one good arm in the air, as if using new toys.

Mrs. Cooke went home, but her baby stayed. A temporary patient identification card was made for the infant, embossed with raised letters, to be used to stamp pages in her chart and label tubes of blood. The ward secretary hadn't yet been informed of a name, and printed the card to read, "Baby Girl Cooke." A pink index card was stamped with this name and glued to the side of her isolation box.

Every hour, her vital signs—blood pressure, pulse, respiratory rate, and temperature—were measured by a nurse. Numbers accumulated to fill yard-long grids of paper. The baby lay hooked up to a bottle of IV fluid that was bigger than she was. Tape covered most of her face, securing an NG tube that brought fluids to her stomach.

My resident helped me to lay out an approach to take with

her parents. I ushered them into a small conference room.

"We decided to name her Valerie," Mrs. Cooke told me. "It was the name of my best friend when I was a little girl. Isn't it a lovely name?"

"Yes. It is."

"I always wanted a little girl. My sister has two children. Hank and I talked for months about having a baby before he finally went along with the idea."

"What's your understanding of her medical status at this point?" I asked.

"She's here now but my husband and I can't wait to take her home."

"How do you feel about the situation?"

"We're going to set the crib up in our bedroom. That way we can watch her."

"What about the difficulties she's had?"

"Oh, I know she has some problems. But the nurse said they would probably be able to help her."

"We're going to try, but we still don't know the extent of the infection or how she will do. She is breathing on her own and her other vital signs have been stable, but we're concerned about her arm. We're going to do some tests to find out what effect the infection might have had."

"I know she won't be going home tomorrow, but we're going to get everything ready, anyway. Hank's buying a crib today."

"It may be very difficult at home."

"Oh no. My mother lives only a few blocks away and can take care of her too."

"I want to emphasize that we need to perform some tests before we know how she's going to do."

A few days later, a CAT scan of the head was performed. A preliminary reading showed that the brain was cluttered with balls that lit up white, representing round cysts of toxoplasma.

I met with the Cookes again. "The preliminary results of the CAT scan are back," I told them. "As you and I discussed before, it's not clear what the prognosis is, but these early results suggest that it's guarded." Mrs. Cooke was silent. "She may have some permanent damage, though the final reading won't be done until tomorrow."

"How long is she going to be here?" Mr. Cooke asked.

"That's hard to say."

"Why don't you buy the crib anyway," Mrs. Cooke told her husband. "That way we'll be all set."

"How are you feeling about this news?" I asked.

"I don't know why this happened," he said slowly and uncomfortably. The sleeves of his plaid lumber shirt were rolled up. His elbows were leaning on his knees.

"These things occur," I said. "Rarely, but they do. I know it is troubling."

"Why did this have to happen to us?"

"What had you been told about the infection before the baby was born?"

"They didn't know what was going to happen," he said. "They thought she might not be born alive."

"But she did okay," Mrs. Cooke added. "And my little baby's going to get through this too."

"I guess we'll just have to do the best we can," he said. "She's still our little girl."

"Let me know if you have any questions. The staff would like to do anything we can to help."

When I told them the official reading of the CAT scan, Mrs. Cooke began to cry. "We don't know fully what this means," I said, "and can't predict how things will go."

"She has the same color hair as my husband's side of the family, you know."

"I'm sure this is upsetting news."

"She's so pretty. She even smiled at me yesterday when I visited. I think she's beginning to recognize me—to know her mama."

"I know this is hard."

"My mother said she would help us out."

"Let me just repeat that we will do everything we can to assist." High-cost technology would be relied on to keep her alive. Because the technology existed that could prolong her life by a few months, it would be employed. It would help the adults involved.

The child was blind from toxoplasmosis, probably deaf, had a lopsided face and couldn't smile, barely moved, and didn't seem to me to respond to other human beings. Mrs. Cooke's difficulty in accepting the infant's impairment was understandable, and it was clear that denial was a major means of coping.

Two days later, Mrs. Cooke arrived carrying a huge corrugated cardboard box in her arms. It was filled with baby toys, all gaily gift-wrapped.

She opened them eagerly. "Here's a pretty bell," she said, smiling at Valerie as she displayed a round plastic toy with a tin bell inside it. The baby lay motionless. Its left arm looked puny. Onto the IV bottle, Mrs. Cooke hooked up a mobile, a white plastic box with four wires protruding from it, on which pink and white knit booties were hung. She wound it up. Tiny metal prongs inside the white box slowly plucked "Twinkle, Twinkle, Little Star."

The song ended. The baby still hadn't moved. The bright wrappings lay scattered on the floor beside Mrs. Cooke. She picked them up and threw them into a garbage bin near the doorway. Several colored plastic bells lay in a cluster in the isolation box.

Mrs. Cooke found it uncomfortable talking to doctors. One of the nurses, Sally Hoyt, lived in the same neighborhood as Mrs. Cooke, and they became friends. Sally was single and loved children. She initially had been taking care of other patients but eventually she traded one of them with another nurse in order to take care of Valerie.

Sally was energetic and friendly. When Mrs. Cooke visited, she often found the nurse feeding Valerie. Sally would sit in one of the wooden rocking chairs placed incongruously between the rows of isolation boxes on the ward. Sally would cradle the infant in her arms and hold a bottle of special formula to her mouth; by then, Valerie was able to drink.

"Valerie slept very well last night," Sally would say as she let the baby gulp down a few more slurps and then patted her on the back. "Isn't that right?" she asked Valerie. "Okay, here's Mommy." She wiped away regurgitated milk that had dribbled onto Valerie's chin. "Yes, sweetheart, I'm going to hand you to Mommy now."

Nobody on the staff ever bothered to change the name on the plastic ID card. The doctors continued to call the patient "Baby Girl Cooke," or sometimes referred to her just as "Cooke." No one talked about sending her home.

Mrs. Cooke walked into the unit more slowly each time she came. As the prognosis grew progressively grimmer, Mrs. Cooke's visits became less frequent. In the weeks that followed, the baby developed other infections, and became ever sicker.

Soon, Mrs. Cooke stopped coming.

In her third month, Baby Girl Cooke died. Sally exchanged a day off with another nurse to attend the small funeral. I had never heard of a nurse or doctor attending a patient's funeral before. Sally went partly as a friend of the family and, I suspect, partly to mourn a child she had known better than anyone else had.

The Unnamed

"What are you doing to my baby?" Mrs. Johnson demanded.

"I'm drawing blood for some routine tests." Her son Claude
appeared more like six months old than his actual one and a
half years. He had come into the hospital severely malnour-
ished, with a history of recurrent infections—earaches, pneumonia, and thrush.

"What are the results?" she asked me the next day.

"They were normal."

"Meaning he won't get any worse?" Her eyes were red. Tears
dried on her cheeks.

"The results showed us that nothing was wrong," I answered.
She appeared relieved. I also arranged with the attending, Dr.
Barber, to test for AIDS, or HTLV III, as it was then called.

Two weeks later, Lou, my resident in pediatrics, two other
interns, two medical students, and I were discussing patients
in hushed tones at the edge of the hallway. Slanted rays of
sunlight filtered in through dusty windows, awakening the shad-

owy ward. The pediatric ward was different from Watkins-9. The atmosphere was brighter. Nurses and doctors expressed their fondness for patients more readily, picking them up and hugging them. "Hey, tiger, what do you have there?" a nurse might greet a patient holding a toy. On the whole, children fare better in the hospital than adults. There are fewer DNRs. Chronic, debilitating diseases are rarer.

But they exist.

Dr. Barber walked up to our huddle. He was tall and slender with curly black hair and wore a yellow button-down shirt and a navy tie with green dinosaurs on it. "The results of the HIV test on the patient Johnson are back," he said. The muscles of his face tightened, and he appeared to be squinting to see something the rest of us were missing. "However, don't forget that as physicians, we are prohibited by law from telling each other or anyone else what the results are, since the procedure was done as part of an experimental protocol, not as a routine test." It was still illegal to get the HTLV III test performed any other way. "Consequently, the results are confidential." He drew in a deep breath. "But, I want you all to think of the implications of the fact that I'm telling you all this."

Lou was unimpressed by Dr. Barber's tone of high secrecy. "I don't get it," he blurted out. "What the hell are you talking about?" He was a tough Italian street kid from Brooklyn, a former public school teacher in a rough neighborhood.

Dr. Barber smiled. "I just want you to think about the fact that I'm telling you that the results are back, though I can't tell you what they are." The attending was trying to say that the AIDS test had come back positive—that the patient had the antibody to the virus floating in his bloodstream, and thus had probably been exposed to AIDS in the past. However, as the test was run as part of a research protocol, the results were not for public consumption, even by those responsible for the patient's care in the hospital.

I entered Claude's room to inform Mrs. Johnson of the diagnosis. She had already whiled away weeks beside him in the hospital.

"I'm afraid I have bad news to report to you, Mrs. Johnson. Our tests show that your son has been exposed to the AIDS virus. I understand this is very upsetting, but we don't yet know what a positive blood test means and whether Claude has the disease or will necessarily get any worse." She wept as I continued to speak. With Kleenex covering her mouth, she nodded, staring at her knees.

Later in the day, I stopped at the room. She was on the phone with her husband, Claude senior. "I can't take it anymore, Claude," she cried, throwing crumpled tissues at the windowsill, which was cluttered with baby bottles, Styrofoam coffee cups, and a pile of Pampers. "I knew they thought he had AIDS. I knew it." She spied me standing near Claude's crib and looked away. I was the unwelcome bearer of bad tidings.

I happened to be on call that evening, and at 8:00 P.M., as I was rushing toward the stairs to handle an emergency on another floor, she approached me.

"I'll be right back and see you in a few minutes," I told her.

"I have to talk to you now," she insisted. "I just have one question."

"Well, okay. What is it?"

"I think something's wrong with him. Can you come look?"

Claude's condition hadn't changed for a few weeks and the nurses hadn't mentioned anything about a change in his status. The patient downstairs was more critically ill. I suspected that she needed help more than her son did at this point.

"I have an emergency downstairs I have to take care of first," I responded. I scurried off, and she skulked away, clearly annoyed. When I saw him later, he was stable.

Claude was given a diagnosis about which no one was allowed to speak, though everyone did. In the minds of nurses and other staff members, he was labeled with a classification applied with increasing frequency in medicine, though not at the time mentioned in the leading medical textbooks—he was diagnosed as "pre-AIDS." He looked merely like a mildly ill child, but it was predicted that he would eventually succumb to the full disease. The term has changed in the past two years to "AIDS-Related Complex." But "pre-AIDS" was a novel term. No other disease was anticipated as sensitively. "Pre-cancer" or "pre-pneumonia" didn't exist as recognized entities. The early stages of most other diseases are conceptualized as part of a continuum, part of a progressive clinical course.

Claude joined another patient on the pediatric ward, Bellevue Stone, who was also believed to have AIDS. The two-and-a-half-year-old orphaned son of a black drug addict mother, he was an ebullient child who didn't look the least bit sick but had been found to have antibodies to the presumed AIDS virus in his blood. A nurse would walk him down the hall each day at the end of a leash tied around his waist. Bellevue—it was rumored that his mother named her offspring after the hospitals in which they were born—usually had much more energy than the fatigued nurse assigned to him for the shift and he would tug her along, running ahead with all his strength. It was unknown whether he was infectious at this clinically benign stage, and no one knew when the virus would begin to sap his strength and cripple his body.

Nurses feared he might spit on or bite other children, though he never did. Not knowing what he might do, what power he possessed to inflict harm, the nurses decided to prevent him from doing anything. He was leashed for walking and otherwise kept in his room with the door shut as he jumped up and down on his crib or bounced a beach ball along the gray tiled floor.

Claude, too, was moved into a private room to isolate him. The nurses would always put on disposable yellow paper gowns before entering. They would wear masks and rubber gloves as well, the cuffs of which they released so far from their skin that the rubber snapped loudly against their wrists. They avoided contact with the gloves as if those films of plastic were somehow contaminated even before being brought into the patient's room.

Lou never wore gowns or masks, however, and rarely gloved up. He trusted the medical literature that ruled out transmission by air or by respiratory secretions. He believed that washing hands with alcohol pads would protect him if his ungloved fingers touched the patient's skin. Lou encouraged the interns to follow his approach.

When Lou and I discussed how to manage Claude's treatment, we referred to his disease as HTLV III. No one on the ward officially uttered the acronym AIDS. Yet everyone knew why Claude was in the hospital. Little by little, people babbled.

One day a Mrs. Stevenson, the mother of another patient, accosted one of the nurses, Dierdra, in the hall. "I've heard there's a patient with AIDS on the floor!" she exclaimed, as if stating that bubonic plague had just wiped out the city. Dierdra fell silent for a moment, weighing what to say. She was twenty-two and had chosen pediatrics because she enjoyed working with children.

Impatient for an answer, Mrs. Stevenson persisted. "Who is it?"

Dierdra explained that it was against established hospital policy for nurses to divulge confidential patient information to anyone outside the patient's family.

Mrs. Stevenson wasn't satisfied. "I no longer want my son to be a patient on this floor," she proclaimed, and stormed off. Later, she cornered me against the cinderblock wall of the hallway. "Which child has AIDS?" she interrogated.

"We usually share patients' diagnoses only with their family," I responded.

"Well," she huffed, "I saw a child drop his bottle in this very hall! The nurse's aide picked it up off the floor and handed it back to him!"

Mrs. Stevenson raved all afternoon and managed to instill fear in other mothers on the ward. The nurses confined Claude even more strictly to his room. He remained strapped in the stroller stationed in the doorway of his cell. He would clutch his bottle to his mouth, gulping formula, and watch with lonely, uncomprehending eyes everyone who passed by.

He saw me as his biggest enemy. I was the one who made him cry by carrying him into the treatment room to draw his blood.

Though cultures of secretions from his lung never grew *Pneumocystis carinii,* he was started on Bactrim and began to improve. I arranged for frequent chest X-rays. I could carry these X-rays on my clipboard, since the films were only the size of his small torso.

Claude's fevers slowly vanished, and a few weeks after starting antibiotics, he went home.

A month later, I saw Mrs. Johnson and Claude on the sidewalk in front of the hospital. She was pushing him along in a blue stroller, his two tiny hands clasping a yellow plastic bottle to his mouth.

"How are you doing?" she asked me. He looked up at me, clenched his bottle tighter, and pushed it closer to his mouth. His eyes widened.

"I'm fine, Mrs. Johnson, how are you and Claude?"

"Oh, we're good. We're just in for a checkup." It was a balmy spring day. Yellow tulips bloomed along the sidewalk. Birds sang. "Come on, Claude," she said. She waved goodbye and pushed him up the driveway toward the hospital's revolving doors.

XXY?

"Come here, Martina," her mother called. The girl sat at the edge of the bed wearing a pink jumper, a white blouse, and black patent leather shoes. Her black hair was gathered back and tied with a gold elastic cord which was threaded through two pink plastic beads, the color of cotton candy. Her legs were crossed at her ankles and were swinging back and forth from the edge of the bed.

"I'm going to have to do a little test," I told her.

Martina Nonez was a six-year-old girl with an inguinal hernia, an outpouching of intestine that had gotten trapped in a canal that plunges from the abdomen into the groin. Such hernias aren't characteristic of females, although they occasionally occur in males in the course of the testicles descending as the fetus develops.

The fact that Martina had a hernia raised the question of whether she was really a female. Were her chromosomes the conventional XX which genetically define her gender? She might possess a different set of these critical genes, perhaps

203

XXY, XO, or even XY—that is, she could be a male whose genetic messages were improperly carried out and resulted in his looking more like a her than a him. Such phenomena exist. To evaluate Martina's genes, a sample of her cells needed to be examined in the lab.

"I need to look inside your mouth," I told her. The most convenient source of tissue is the inside cheek, known as the buccal mucosa. The outer, epithelial cells lining the mouth flake off frequently, and readily replace each other as front line defenses against any unwelcome matter that enters the mouth. These cells are flat and wide, so that relatively few are needed to tile the inner surface of the oral cavity. Their size also makes them ideal candidates for study. Unusually accessible, they can be harvested simply by wiping a wooden tongue depressor along the inside of the cheek.

"Open up wide," I urged. She stretched open her lips.

"Ahhhh," she said as if I were a dentist. I touched the edge of the wooden blade to the inside of her mouth. She got ready to whimper, looking pleadingly to her mother for rescue in the event of danger. I swiftly drew the stick along the wet pink wall of her cheek. She knit her brow and looked up at me in perplexed fright.

"All done!" I exclaimed. "That wasn't too bad now, was it?" She didn't answer. I transferred the wet glop onto two glass microscope slides, neatly wrapped up my prizes in a brown paper towel, and said goodbye.

I went up to the cytology laboratory. It was relegated to the top floor of the hospital tower, practically the attic. The windows were dingy with decades of dirty rain splatter, making them opaque. Vague shapes of the city's skyline were barely discernible through the panes. It was a place where all eyes squinted into microscope lenses and rarely peeked outside.

In the front lab room, bowls of colored dyes stood in neat

rows on a bench. Funnels lined with paper filters sprouted from the mouths of bottles. The dyes—fluorescent orange, rich magenta, and Prussian blue—had formed colored concentric rings as they had been spilled through the filters, painting the paper. With hearts of bright orange or deep red, and outer edges tinged with pure white paper untouched by the dye, the paper funnels resembled flowers blooming in a row along the ebony lab bench.

The lab technician led me to a microscope, where she showed me the cells from a smear. "We count the percentage of Barr bodies we see in the nuclei of cells," she explained. "The cells of females have two X chromosomes, one of which is superfluous and crumples up into a clump discarded onto the side of the nuclei. This means that female cells can be identified by the presence of these dark blots, or 'Barr bodies,' at the edge of the nuclei. However, the Barr body is not always visible or perhaps even present.

"If seven percent or more of the cells have Barr bodies, then we say the person is female," she continued. "If it's one percent or less, we call the person male. There's a gray area in between," she explained.

"What do you do then?" I inquired.

"We go ahead and do a much more complicated, precise chromosome count."

Even at this sophisticated laboratory, there was a hazy, indeterminate range of results. The more advanced test might also leave room for doubt.

The final lab results might suggest that Martina would more appropriately have been a boy; or that, to remain female, she would eventually need to be surgically cut, patched, and sewn up.

The knowledge that she was less of a girl than had been suspected could also be inconsequential. Some of an organism's characteristics are determined directly by his or her genes, and are said to constitute his or her "genotype." Other features, resulting from contrasting genes blending together, or from genes expressing themselves imperfectly (often due to environmental interference), are referred to as one's "phenotype." Martina's phenotype had made her genitalia look more like a girl's than a boy's. Nature makes mistakes, however, and vast room exists for variation. Anatomy is sculpted by genes, but in the workshop of the cell, every work of art differs from the next. The variations are usually subtle, but can be significant enough to confuse the model and the final product.

Even if I discovered that she was not a pure female, that she should have been named Martin instead of Martina, I wouldn't advise changing the gender already assigned her. She would always be a girl because she had been brought up until now thinking she was.

Endocrinologists—hormone experts—whom I could call in might opt to remake her to conform to her sex more closely if they thought that discrepancies might become more pronounced. Plastic surgery might be implemented if she were found to be genetically a male, or mistakenly have a male chromosome that would shape her genitalia ambiguously. Her anatomy might begin to differ too far from the classic female, and sluggishly rest in between male and female when the age of puberty arrived with its demand for commitment to one side or the other of the gender divide. Plastic surgeons could ensure that she continued to look as much like a female as possible as she grew older. But if she didn't have the full reproductive anatomy of her sex at birth, they wouldn't be able to provide her with one now. Outward appearances were one thing, but complex inner organs, the tools of creating new members of the species, were something even doctors couldn't supply. We could touch her up but not remake her.

Even if nature had erred in her artistry, Martina wouldn't find out, at least not now. I might not even trouble her parents with these disturbing questions.

Martina was taken to the operating room for repair of her hernia. Then she rested. She was unaware that anyone doubted her sex. She didn't know why she was in the ward. But since her mother was there also, it didn't occur to her to ask. Her mother had bought her a new doll just for coming to the hospital. The doll had braids which Martina wanted too, now, instead of pulling her hair to the back of her head.

Martina liked being with her mother all the time in the ward. Mrs. Nonez slept on a big armchair with a matching stool. Martina thought it was better than nursery school, where she wouldn't see her mother until returning home for lunch.

But some things in the hospital scared her. After the operation, she romped around the hall wearing yellow frilly dresses, yellow stockings, and white anklet socks folded over at the top. She peered queerly at the other kids, who vaguely didn't seem right to her, different from the kids in her class at school. They wore pajamas all day and some looked puny. She rarely spoke to the other children and didn't know what they did. Did they live here while she was only visiting? No one told her.

A few days after I had taken Martina's cells to the lab, the results arrived back on the ward. The computer printout sheet didn't reveal what percentage of her cells contained Barr bodies. But it confirmed, in dot-matrix computer type, that she carried two sex chromatids, both XX, and that she was, in their estimation, a girl. I was glad she would be staying the way she was. She'd be glad, too, if she knew.

The Seven Dwarfs

W anda Mayson was born with a defective liver. Five years
ago, she would have lived for as long as it held out,
her body a time bomb. But experimental liver transplants had
been performed in adults, and recently in children, and her
doctor decided to make her one of the first child recipients of
someone else's liver. She was launched on what was to become
a long series of hospitalizations for surgery and for close monitoring of any ache or abnormal liver enzymes. Her parents
hoped the transplant would help her. As she was only six years
old, she had no say in the matter.

In the pediatric ward, Wanda would sit on a red metal wagon
and be pushed along by two other patients, boys whom she
had befriended. She knew the ropes of the ward better than
they did, even though her two companions were older, aged
nine and eleven. Age didn't matter. What drew them to her
was her courage.

Each day on morning rounds, as the doctors traveled from
room to room, visiting all the patients, Wanda would sit in her

cart several doors ahead of our group and watch. When we progressed down the hallway toward her, she would direct her two friends to push the cart along in the same direction, keeping a safe distance ahead of what must have seemed to her a great white wave. Lou would pick up the pace. "Faster! Faster!" she'd cry to her two male drivers, banging her hand on the side of the cart. We'd speed up, holding our stethoscopes in front of us so they wouldn't knock against our stomachs. Wanda would slap the metal wagon still more excitedly. The two boys were soon speeding her cart down the hallway, the medical staff jogging after her, specialists and attending physicians in the lead, followed by Lou and others of the house staff. Medical students and nurses brought up the rear. The nurse Dierdra whirled along a rack of medical charts.

The pediatrics ward was a noisy circus. Wanda raced past the nursing station, where children of different shapes and sizes wandered by or were parked in strollers, barred in metal cribs, or stranded in wheelchairs. A child in a stroller was banging and shrieking to attract the attention of a nearby nurse who was trying to do her paper work. Danny, a two-foot-tall boy, dragged a six-foot-long stuffed yellow banana through the hall on a leash as Wanda sailed by. A curious toddler was becoming aware of the IV pole three times his height to which he was attached. The pole crashed to the floor as he dragged it along, testing its limits of balance. One baby in a crib wrestled with newly found external objects—his legs, which kept getting in his way as he tried to roll over.

Wanda's entourage was nearing the double metal doors that barred the end of the hallway. The doors opened on air suction hinges controlled by special buttons high above her head. Her companions glanced back in fear as we approached.

The cart slowed down, and was then besieged. "We have to take a look at you, Wanda," Lou said. It was necessary to evaluate her each day to assess her clinical status. Since this was a teaching floor, students examined her, too, as part of their training. She strained to escape, but couldn't see past the white coats huddled around her. The two boys were swept away, leaving her alone. Strange hands probed up her shirt and slid down her collar, pressed her tummy, and tapped on her back. Hands and white sleeves and cold metal stethoscopes swarmed around her. "No," she cried, still sitting up, thrashing her hands noisily on the sides of her cart in anger.

"It will just take a minute," Lou told her. The hands continued. She cried. Then the crowd finished and went away, going on to the next patient, leaving her clothes disheveled, her companions banished. I lagged behind to pull her shirt back down over the top of her small body. "Don't cry, you're okay," I said.

Throughout the ward and above her head, bright cartoon characters were pasted to the walls. Across the hall from her room were Snow White and the Seven Dwarfs glued onto the dull yellow paint. But the cartoon characters on the walls didn't mirror the blood and Betadine faced by those trapped on the ward. The Mylar balloons brought as gifts by visitors and tied to cribs and strollers reflected back the warped and colorless shapes of the ward. Wanda was a jaded veteran of hospitals, wise to the ways of these institutions. She had wide eyes, charming and intriguing. But she knew that the pediatric floor was not the homey playground that nurses and doctors tried hard to intimate.

The transplant she had received might give her only three or four more years of life. Probably no more. Her doctors had undertaken this costly investment as a carefully monitored trial. They chose as their laboratory the body of this beautiful and innocent little girl. I admired her bravery in running from and defying us as we tampered with her body. But we had created a monster. Wanda would never be a normal child. We had spoiled her. She felt abused. Her fierce grimaces expressed her rage and masked her utter helplessness. She had been medicated with steroids to slow her body from attacking the foreign liver, and the drug had produced side effects, fattening her cheeks, flattening out her face to give her what was termed "moon facies," and adding a lump of fat to the nape of her neck, making her resemble a hunchback. Patches of short hairs had sprouted in odd places on her body—for instance, her upper back. The medicines and procedures had stunted her growth, aging her face and transforming her child's body into that of a midget.

Her two brothers hated coming to the hospital, and often remained home when their mother stayed with Wanda. They rarely saw her. Now Mrs. Mayson didn't sleep overnight in the lounge chair and footstool as often as she had in the initial stages of her daughter's illness and treatment. Wanda's condition was labeled chronic now, not acute.

Wanda began to recognize me. I smiled and greeted her when I saw her on the ward. One afternoon, I was called to draw her blood. I dreaded having to hurt her, and I knew I was about to be added to her list of evil doctors.

Blood from children is usually drawn not in their rooms but in a special treatment room, so that patients will dissociate the trauma of this procedure from the security of their own niches. Dierdra and another nurse carried her into the windowless treatment room. They lifted her onto a table, laid her down, and held her there.

"How are you doing today, Wanda?" I said. She peered at me suspiciously, then turned her head away. "I'm going to have to draw a little bit of blood from you, honey." I tried to fill my voice with sympathy. She kept her head staunchly averted. "It'll only take a second." She was not persuaded.

She remained aloof, scornful, barely glancing at me from the corner of her eye.

This business was going to be traumatic for both of us. The four of us were going to have to work something out. "I know it's not nice but we have to do it."

I had ceased carrying blood-drawing equipment with me. I took some needles and syringes from boxes, and pulled a metal stool along the tiled floor to the table where she lay. She watched me from the corner of her eye.

Then she mechanically extended her elbow, exposing her soft inner arm to the needle.

I was awed. She resigned herself to blood drawing unflinchingly. Smarter and more discriminating than I had imagined, she knew that one doctor taking blood from her was necessary, but that fifteen of them jabbing her tender belly with cold metal stethoscopes every day weren't helping her.

"Thank you, Wanda," I said after filling the tubes with blood.

"You're welcome," she replied in a meek voice. She jumped down from the table by herself, refusing the offer of a hand. Wanda strode toward the door in big steps and marched out into the corridor. She looked one way and then the other for her friends and galloped down the hall.

Brodsky

L ou and I traveled from room to room on midnight rounds.
I carried a clipboard that held the sign-out sheets handed
to me by my fellow interns before they had departed for the
day. We came to Room 618, which is outfitted with four cribs.

"Who's in here?" Lou whispered so as not to wake them,
whoever they were.

I riffled through the crinkled sheets of paper stained with
coffee, iodine antiseptic soap, and blood.

"Brodsky," I mumbled back to him.

"Yup! Over here!" we heard an excited voice shout from the
crib in the far right corner.

Lou and I glanced at each other, perplexed, and headed in
its direction. This ward was full of infants and toddlers. The
confident and mature voice rang incongruously through the
darkened room of barred beds.

When we reached the siderails, I was shocked. An attractive
face grinned at me. Her head was normal sized for a teen-
ager, but the distance from her neck to her toes couldn't have

been more than two feet. She was tinier than a midget, who's at least adult-proportioned, though child-sized.

"Are you Brodsky?" I asked, amazed.

"That's me!" she exclaimed. "My name's Lisa."

Her hair was stylishly cut, closely cropped on the sides, and she wore sickle-shaped earrings and soft makeup. She wasn't one of my patients. I was caring for her only that night. But I was confused by her.

I turned back to my wrinkled sign-out sheets to find out why she was in the hospital. "Sixteen-year-old female with osteogenesis imperfecta," it read, a rare genetic bone disease, "now with pneumonia. Today is day 3 of a 7-day course of antibiotics." No one had warned me about her appearance. Perhaps she was too odd and disturbing to describe. She suffered multiple bone fractures, growth retardation, and progressive skeletal deformity. She was bedbound and her bones hadn't enlarged sufficiently to allow expulsion of air effective enough to cleanse her lungs. She was vulnerable to pulmonary infections, a "setup," as doctors termed it, because of her constricted chest.

I think of the brain as the most important human organ. When I dissected a cadaver, I proceeded up the body toward the head, sawing it open last. I conceived of the other organs— the heart, kidneys, and lungs—as supports that kept the brain nourished and alive. Lisa was almost all brain.

On evening rounds, we made final checks on the sleeping rooms. I would have to listen to her heart and lungs. I warmed the cold metal stethoscope in my hand. Metal chills warm, unexpecting flesh. Her head lay sunken on a pillow looking up at the ceiling. Her neck appeared too thin to turn her comparatively massive head readily, making it necessary for her to stare straight forward. Perhaps it was easier for her to keep her eyes focused narrowly on what lay ahead and be blind to the expressions of others as they glimpsed her from the side.

I lifted the sheet a few inches to place my stethoscope in order to hear her lungs, instructing her to breathe in and out through her mouth. Then I moved the bell farther down her body to listen to her heart.

My hand held the sheet over the upper part of her body. She was smiling at the sky. Before the sheet settled back down over her torso it billowed upward a few inches.

"There," I said. She was well used to invasions of stethoscopes, needles, and doctors.

In adjusting the cover, I had noted the presence of pubic hair. The disease had no impact on the neurological or endocrine systems. Only her bones. They alone had stunted her. She was not merely all brain. She was a sexual creature as well.

"Any problems with her?" Lou asked.

"No. Not tonight."

"Status quo," Lou concluded.

I never commented on her deformity or development to the rest of the staff, nor did they say anything about it to me.

I didn't inquire further about her. At this point in the year, I separated knowledge that was necessary, relevant to my care of patients, from what was unessential. If further details were needed, I could always obtain them from a patient's chart. I had also come to use a patient's old medical chart more, to place a patient's current problems in the context of their past hospitalizations and their "history," as the story of a patient's medical problems over time was termed.

I never had cause to read her chart. The night was busy and internship would be over in a few days.

The next morning, on the elevator I took to the ward, an overweight Hassidic man shuffled about in the corner. His moist hand wrung the tassles of a white silk shawl. He looked as if he were heading to Poland in the last century. An hour later, wearing his prayer shawl, he was standing at the foot of her bed gently rocking back and forth, bowing before her, chanting prayers, while holding a small worn black book in his pale hands. He didn't stop when I walked by the room.

She was a high school student, and her friends from school visited her on the ward. They wheeled her up and down the corridor in a baby carriage, chatting.

Occasionally, her stroller would be parked by the nursing station. "Hi, how are you?" she greeted everyone who passed. I thought of a popular adage among the nursing staff on the pediatric ward: the nicest people get the worst diseases. The aphorism was invoked whenever a child more innocent and beautiful than most, whose parents were well liked by the staff, was being tested for cancer or a disabling disease. An accepted corollary was that children and parents who were obstreperous would turn out to be disease free.

A few days later, I spotted Lisa as she was about to be discharged. Her carriage was parked by the nursing station. She was beaming at the air. A family member was no doubt making the final arrangements for her departure.

"So, you're going home?"

"Yes."

"Are you planning on returning to school at all soon?"

"I sure am. I'm excited about getting back," she answered from her stroller.

"I saw your friends visiting you the other day."

Her eyes lit up. "Yes. They came after school. They're wonderful." She was the most enthusiastic patient I had ever known, the most loving and accepting of life with its peculiar hardships.

She didn't seem to perceive anything incongruous, displaying not the least sign of lack of confidence, embarrassment, or recognition that she was extraordinary. She didn't acknowledge that an observer might be surprised. The absence of such a reaction was striking. She appeared not to be bothered by the disease.

I wanted to ask her how she did it—what kept her going? Her strength was not promoted by doctors and medicine. Physicians could give her drugs, but nothing to infuse her with a sense of purpose. It may have been that her enthusiasm had come from her Hassidic family and community, from the mere fact of her survival, as well as from herself. She retained her spirit not because of us but despite us. I had no life-affirming inspirations to offer her in dealing with her illness, no sustaining images that she didn't already possess, nothing to foster courage. The only symbols of hope I offered were medicine and drugs, which were necessary but not sufficient. Her family reading prayer healed her spirit more than anything I could provide.

Discharge
with Medical Advice

M y last night on call began on a Friday evening. I admitted
a patient at 6:00 A.M. as the light of the sky was just
beginning to brighten the windows. Morning was approaching.
Out of the distant blackness, the pale shapes of the city began
to materialize. With them would arrive a hospital full of staff,
including other doctors to replace me and be responsible for
the lives I had guarded for the night.

Saturday morning, my internship ended. I was glad it was
over, relieved it was behind me. I had aged by more than one
year. In the past, people saw suffering and death when they
were sent off to war. The closest I had come was this year.
Never again would I report to an office routinely one morning
out of every three to sign death certificates.

The last thirty-six hours had been noteworthy for how un-
remarkable they were. The level of anxiety I felt at the beginning of the year when on call never fully dissipated. I had
heard in the past of interns uncorking bottles of champagne
on the hospital roof on their final morning, but as an intern

now, I neither saw nor heard any such hoopla. Mostly I was sleepy and knew that the second year of residency would soon start. A rookie would struggle with the tragedies I was now deserting. There was no call for celebration.

One year ago, I had graduated from medical school. The only meaningful portion of the commencement ceremony was an optional recitation of the Hippocratic oath. The conferring of degrees in a yellow and white circus tent on the medical school dormitory lawn had little impact on me. The only way in which that ritual had changed my identity was the adding of two letters after my name.

But internship was different.

What I learned during the year was no great single revelation, no prescription for revamping American medicine. Rather, I saw how individuals offered fleeting glimpses of themselves, how they dealt with disease and death, and strove to piece together shards of the familiar in this otherwise sterile environment. I had become less idealistic, and felt less distanced from other people's pain than I had been as a student. I had seen that medicine is not always a science. Many things were done as part of the art, or because of tradition, convenience, or the availability of resources. Interns accomplished a lot of good, curing countless patients and comforting friends and families. But successful outcomes were viewed as if they were universal. They were not. Many patients I saw lingered in the hospital, close to dying. In medical education, one learns first, while in anatomy class, from the dead; then, during internship, from the dying, and the sickest. Not until a resident would I spend most of my time with outpatients, who were the healthiest and could be treated while at home.

I had come to see myself as a doctor and had begun to feel more confident in that role, accepting its pains and its perks.

One day near the end of the year, I had missed lunch and

was hurrying through the lobby past the gift shop. I decided to buy a present for myself—a chocolate bar. The woman behind the counter in a pink hospital smock dawdled, making neat piles of paper bags, ignoring me. I stood there for several minutes. "Here's the money," I said finally, pushing it toward her on the counter.

"You have to wait until I ring it up."

"Yes, but I'm in a hurry."

"Who do you think you are?"

"I'm a doctor," I said in my white coat, "and I have patients to take care of." I deposited my money on the counter and walked off.

Walt Simmons had been counting down the last one hundred days before a new intern would liberate him. "I decided to say goodbye to my patients," he told me one day during our last week. "But they're all either demented, comatose or dying. It's sad. Few of my cancer patients were ever in a hospital before a year and a half ago. Most have come in several times since then. Many will probably be dead within a year."

In this feat of human technology called a hospital, part of the official procedure was moving on. I had gotten to know and like many of the patients and nurses. But I probably wouldn't see them again either.

At 7:30 Saturday morning, a woman in a clean white coat approached me in the nursing station.

"Are you the resident?" she asked.

"No. I'm the intern."

"But you look so calm. I thought you must be a resident. I'm Tina Whalin. I'm picking up your service. I don't begin until tomorrow, but I decided to come in a day early to hear about the patients directly from you, if that's okay."

"No problem," I said, introducing myself. "You'll be better

prepared. Have a seat." I grinned as I pulled out a sign-out sheet from my clipboard, describing each of my patients. "How does it feel to be starting?"

"I'm not sure," she said. "It's funny being back in a hospital. I've spent the past week, since graduating from medical school, vacationing up in Vermont with my boyfriend."

"It's good you were able to get away. Internship starts up quickly and becomes all-consuming. Shall we go over the patients?" She nodded and I placed the sheet of paper between us on the counter in front of us.

"The first one is Stacy Tomley. History number 4102639. She's an eight-year-old white female BIBA with a . . ."

"What's BIBA?"

"Brought in by ambulance."

"I've never seen that before. I'll have to remember it." She removed a pocket-sized loose-leaf notebook from her white coat and jotted down the acronym.

I didn't remember first hearing or using this expression, but I had come to take it for granted. I continued to tell her about the patient.

"Any other questions?" I asked after describing the last case on the list, and handing her the paper.

"No . . . not really." She hesitated. "But how was it?"

"What do you mean?"

"Being an intern. I just want to survive it. I keep telling myself that in one year it'll be over." She laughed. I must have been timorous my first day, too, or should have been. Some students dove into medical school and internship knowing exactly what to expect. Others dealt with the uncertainty in different ways. In retrospect, I had showed up the first day knowing less than I thought, and was unsure of what to anticipate. My responses were less hardened as a result. "Did you learn a lot?" she asked.

"Yes, an incredible amount."

"How would you sum up the year?"

How could I describe my experiences, all that I had seen and heard?

We talked for a few minutes, but I was done for the year and eager to leave. I shook her hand and walked off toward the elevator bank.

I had arrived in the hospital thirty-six hours earlier. After a night on call, no one bid me "thank you" for my toil. Now, no one said goodbye.

My mind was drained, and I felt weak. My legs barely held up my body. I walked into the white sunlight outside and gazed at people strolling up and down the sidewalk, looking healthy and free from IV poles. Familiar yellow taxicabs hurtled down the street uncaring. I had forgotten that the world still existed outside. I was surprised to see it, fresh, again.

EPILOGUE:
Terra Incognita

At one point during my internship, I cared for a patient named Charlotte Row. A pleasant elderly woman, she had a four-month history of progressive dementia, and had recently developed a tremor, and an inability to remember things she was told, where she was, or where she had placed things. These are symptoms to which anyone might fall prey, especially if tired, fretful, or old. But Mrs. Row soon was forgetting her daughters' names and the location of the bathroom in her own apartment. She began laughing without provocation, even when serious matters were discussed. Her local doctor assumed her diagnosis was Alzheimer's disease.

But then Mrs. Row developed delusions that her family was going to kill her. I saw her, collected a history, and performed a careful physical exam. Dr. Spencer, a professor of Neurology, listed the possible diagnoses, from the most common and likely, to the "zebras," as exotic diseases are dubbed. At the top of the list was Alzheimer's, followed by multi-infarct dementia, and near the end, Pick's disease and Creutzfeldt-Jakob disease.

Standard blood tests measuring electrolytes, thyroid function, and Vitamin B were all normal. I sent Mrs. Row for a Computerized Tomographic Scan, a three-dimensional X-ray of her brain, which also turned out okay. To help sort out the problem, I "tapped her," that is, performed a spinal tap, or as doctors describe it to patients, a lumbar puncture. I painted the loose dry skin of her back with brown soap. My gloved thumb kneaded her back, feeling for a soft spot in the bony grid protecting her spinal cord. I lanced her skin with a thin needle, and squeezed it into her muscle, sliding it between the scooped notches of her vertebrae, aiming toward her navel. My finger felt a quiet pop, transmitted through the metal probe. As I slipped a thin wire out of the hollow bevel, clear watery spinal fluid dripped out. The liquid filled several test tubes, which I labeled, packaged in plastic bags, and sent off for tests.

The studies yielded normal results. Meanwhile, she worsened. Her body began to spasm in brief, irregular tremors. I ordered an electroencephalogram, or EEG, a graph of her brain waves. The needles shivered nervously across the spool of paper, which is normal, but they periodically burst into frenzy, signifying one of several illnesses. Her clinical "presentation" helped narrow the list. I finally concluded that she had Creutzfeldt-Jakob disease.

I had seen such an ailment before.

Several years earlier, the year prior to entering medical school, I had worked in Papua New Guinea, studying the epidemiology of the neurological disease kuru. This disease of the brain, caused by a family of germs termed "slow unconventional viruses," leads to dementia and, ultimately, death.

Kuru was first charted medically by Dr. D. Carleton Gajdusek. Much of his youth had been spent hiking in the woods with a biologist aunt of his, overturning stones to observe the species of worms squiggling away and lichens and fungi blossoming underneath in the dark. He studied physics before medicine, and at the age of twenty-nine, found himself in Australia at the Eliza Hall Institute in the laboratory of Sir McFarlane Burnet, who had won the Nobel Prize a few years earlier for his own medical research. But Carleton's lab was to be beyond the walls of any building. He traveled to the remote island of New Guinea, lying to the north of Australia, in search of new diseases. For him, the island was one vast natural lab.

Once there, he began hearing reports of a strange disease affecting isolated tribes in the Eastern Highlands. Only one physician was working in the region, Dr. Vincent Zigas. Zigas was as drawn to the exotic as Gajdusek. Born in Estonia in 1920, he was educated in Lithuania and Germany and had to fulfill his quest to become a physician by studying in the medical facilities of Nazi Germany. He was romantic and idealistic, and was revolted by the terrors of the war and the postwar upheaval in Germany and Eastern Europe. He chose to forgo his ties to his homeland and he escaped to Australia, only to find that his medical degree wasn't honored there. Though disappointed, he discovered that he would be eligible to practice in the colony of New Guinea. He opted to serve there and survive as best he could. There he stayed, a lone German in the primitive jungle, penetrating farther and farther into the hinterland, healing the sick as well as he could, and befriending natives. He was the first physician to ever see kuru.

When Gajdusek arrived in 1956, he found Zigas, who took him to see cases of this disease. Gajdusek observed that the disease crippled primarily children and women and affected only certain tribes. The two physicians began traveling through the region on foot to map out the boundaries of the epidemic. Much of the area was still labeled as "uncontrolled" by the government and listed on maps as "uncharted," or *terra incognita*.

Gajdusek returned to the United States and began the second phase of his investigation, bringing kuru into the laboratory. He shipped back with him brains gathered on autopsy. He inoculated animals intracerebrally by injecting infected brain tissue into their skulls. He used chimps and squirrel monkeys, guinea pigs, baboons, gorillas, and mice. Most infectious diseases take a few days to attack their host. Gajdusek watched carefully. But nothing happened. The animals remained stubbornly healthy. Colleagues urged him to give up. The disease must be genetic, not infectious, they argued. But Gajdusek waited. Weeks slipped by uneventfully, then months. Still his menagerie ate, ran, and frolicked.

But ten months later, one of the chimps began behaving peculiarly, licking and eating in bizarre ways. The animal began to show the equivalent of neurological deficits observed in New Guineans.

Over the subsequent months, much of this colony of primates displayed symptoms and died from the disease. Initially, only those animals that had been infected subcutaneously, intravenously, or directly in the brain developed the ailment, not those who had been fed the material by mouth. But later, direct consumption was found to be contagious too.

A whole new family of infectious agents was discovered, termed "slow unconventional viruses." Gajdusek considered other names. He pondered whether the agent was similar to viroids, which attack plants, or should be christened with a new term, such as "virin." Another researcher, Stanley Pruisner, has since suggested the name "prion," for protein, which he believes is the major constituent of the particle itself.

Gajdusek sought other diseases that might be related to kuru. He discovered that Creutzfeldt-Jakob disease (CJD) can be transmitted by a virus, similar to the one that causes kuru, but that CJD can also occur spontaneously, without any known exposure, and kills one person per million each year throughout the world. Roughly two hundred people in the United States die of the disease each year, recently among them the choreographer George Balanchine.

The genes of the virus may be able to insert themselves into human chromosomes, where they sit quietly, silently passed from one generation to the next until some unknown triggering event occurs, forcing the invader's genes to pop out of the chromosome, become copied, and instigate disaster. Laboratories around the world are investigating this unique process.

Gajdusek surmised that a member of the Fore tribe had probably died in the past of Creutzfeldt-Jakob disease. Isolated cases of CJD have been reported in New Guinea. The Fore tribe is cannibilistic. When one of its members die, his or her loved ones consume the body. As one anthropologist put it, the tribesmen's cemeteries were their stomachs. Gajdusek hypothesized that a Fore tribesman with CJD was consumed at a cannibalistic feast, exposing others to the virus. The participants at this feast were themselves later eaten, and an epidemic gradually spread.

Twenty-five years ago, the practice of cannibalism was extinguished by Westerners, but the virus can take that long before compromising its host, hence the term "slow virus." The last cases of kuru were still living among the Fore, though their numbers were rapidly diminishing.

The more that has been learned about kuru, the more CJD has become a mystery. Do humans in every corner of the globe carry the virus in their genes as a stowaway, waiting to slip out? If so, how did the virus distribute itself in this way in the first place? Is it a normal part of our genes gone berserk? How many other diseases are caused by viruses sneaking along in our chromosomes?

I was fortunate to work at Gajdusek's lab at the National Institutes of Health while I was in college. When I graduated, an interesting problem was presenting itself in New Guinea. Though the number of patients had dwindled, pockets of cases were emerging sporadically. After a few years of no cases, a village would suddenly find three young men succumbing to symptoms within a few months of each other and dying of the disease all within a year. What was the cause of this strange clustering of patients? Were these cases the result of the last feasts held in each village?

Did the virus possess the heretofore unknown property of being able to lie dormant in the bodies of different people for decades and then spring suddenly into action virtually simultaneously in these different hosts? To answer these questions, I would have to travel to New Guinea. My mission would answer these questions and have another purpose as well.

In recent years, many tribesmen who felt a headache or stomachache feared they had been stricken with kuru. Their fellow villagers, all of whom had watched mothers and siblings die of the disease, shared these terrors. I was sent by the NIH to differentiate current patients from psychosomatic cases in order to elucidate the epidemiology and to measure its incubation periods.

I also went out of a sense of wanderlust. I had read Conrad's *Lord Jim* in my last semester of college, and was inspired by images of rich experiences in the distant tropics.

My destination was the Eastern Highlands, home of the Fore. I flew into the capital, Port Moresby, unconnected by roads to any other part of the country. No road leaves the city to travel more than seventy miles before halting in dense tropical rain forest. The first leg of my journey was flying to the coastal port of Lae. From there, I would drive up the one major roadway on the island, the Highlands Highway.

The Highway slithered over the fingers of mountain ranges rising up from the plains, pulling me into another world. Behind lay the coastal plain, flat, green, and Westernized. Ahead stretched the dense and still largely uncharted rain forests of the Highlands. In there, somewhere, lived the world's last great concentration of primitive peoples. Until the 1930s, Westerners had believed that the interior was uninhabited. No white men had ever been there. I looked back over my shoulder and rarely glanced far ahead. I didn't know where I was going except the name of my next destination, the town of Goroka, the last frontier post of the Eastern Highlands.

The town of Goroka has the feel of the old American West, the excitement and essential loneliness of the frontier. The town supports a handful of bars, two for whites and a half-dozen for natives, one dance hall/disco run by missionaries, at which no alcohol is served, two trading posts, a bakery, and a hotel. At the central crossroads, throngs of mountain tribesmen, in for a day of barter and amusement, mingle with their urban counterparts. The former, wearing traditional dress, are naked but for a few discreetly positioned leaves or strings of beads. Most walk barefoot, their dusty feet padding along the earthen roads.

From Goroka I left for the village of Waisa. The road that led to it was most readily passable. The town was originally laid out above a river, with small clusters of huts scattered down to the river's edge. When the "road" had been graded in the 1950s, the villagers had moved their huts up the hill to be closer to this artery. Their ancestors had lived on the same piece of land for several millenia, but there was no evidence that man had populated the place for more than a decade. No building stood longer than five years. That's how long it took the thatched bamboo huts to rot. There were no signs that a past had ever existed. History, in Waisa, was what could be conveyed by the tongues of the elders. Except for the yearly passing of Christmas, whose celebration has recently been imposed by missionaries, there is no sense of time that extends further back than a hazy few days. To say "two years ago," one says in pidgin, "Bifo tupela Krismas," derived from the English, "before two Christmases." In the traditional local language, the term for "three days ago" is synonymous with the word for "the past," and the word for "three days from now" also means "the future."

I had arrived in Waisa in the middle of the rainy season. Each afternoon, the mountains were lashed by angry rain squalls. But the mornings were hot and dry, and by ten o'clock the sun had baked the bread-colored ground to a crisp.

Accompanied by three native guides, I prepared to set out on foot to see my first patient in another hamlet, named Agatasa, which bordered on largely uncharted forests stretching hundreds of miles to the island's southern coast. It was here that the practice of cannibalism had persisted the longest.

I started walking up a path away from my hut when I was approached by three or four elderly men, garbed only in native dress of leaves around their waist. One was carrying a hand-made bow and arrow. They began to talk to me. "My God, these people are cannibals," I suddenly thought, "these men whom I have befriended and into whose hands I have trustingly placed myself." I had somehow suppressed whatever moral repugnance I might have had to their having engaged in this practice. I was surprised at how far this fact had receded behind my need to cooperate with them in order to survive.

As I proceeded on my journey into the "bush," as the tropical rain forest is called, the heat rapidly began to take its toll. My mouth was soon as dry as a cracked gourd. My legs churned like unoiled machine parts on the stubborn ground. The birds fell silent. Leaves drooped.

But then the trail slipped under the cool green canopy of rain forest. I felt the relief of mud sloshing underfoot and welcomed the ripe, juicy vines that draped down. We passed a niche where a waterfall dashed out, fresh and delicious. I washed, drenching myself, and slaked my thirst in the shady cave of ferns and trees. The stream bubbled, trickled, and sluiced around me in miniature cataracts and aqueducts. I stood beneath the waterfall until I was completely soaked. Within minutes back on the sunlit trail, I was again dry, but refreshed.

I finally reached the hamlet which was to be my base for collecting data for several days. I was hosted in the best native hut in the village, built on the village's highest hill and accessible only by crossing a treacherous hillside of clay. I slipped several times in my ascent as I clawed at the oily red mud, greasing my hands, knees and boots.

These Stone Age villages were not graced with idyllic calm. Life was hard and barren, the diet impoverished and limited to beans, tasteless yams, and tall green stalks called *pitpit*, which, when cooked and stripped of outer sheaths, revealed a fleshy core that tasted, to my surprise, like asparagus. Other staples were more insipid. I had been forewarned about the lack of herbs or spices used in Stone Age cooking. I'd armed myself with a bottle of curry powder, but never expected what I found. At my first native meal, I sprinkled the yellow specks over the top of a bulky potato, and took a bite. The food was dry, tasteless, and difficult to swallow. I spread the powder thickly over the next portion. Again the food was as unpalatable as wood. I heaped on a mound of the powder and its aroma began at last to cover up the dense blandness. Almost my entire bottle of spice was spent on one meal. I had never realized the extent to which vegetables in the West, even those as relatively dull as potatoes, have been scientifically hybridized to enhance their flavor.

At dinner everyone took yams and vegetables, wrapped in banana leaves, and sat off alone. There were no tables or chairs. Little was said by way of dinner-time conversation. Eating was also segregated by the sexes, the men venturing further away from the *mumu,* the pit in which the vegetables were steamed. After a day of speaking only pidgin, my head ached from my inability to communicate my thoughts and feelings in this limited language.

The first night I sat on the floor of the bamboo hut, transcribing my field notes into a notebook by the light of a Coleman oil lamp I had brought. The entire village turned out to watch. They gaped silently as I performed the heretofore unseen process of writing. Theirs was an unwritten language. They didn't possess paper, and some had never seen a lamp.

The hut was cramped and leaky. But eventually, I curled up to sleep in a blanket I had brought. A few hours later, I was to awaken when the house began to shake. I rose, convinced someone was sawing the structure down at its stilts. In the bright moonlight, two pigs (they were half wild boar) were heaving themselves back and forth against the structure's supports, scraping fleas off their skin. I went back to sleep as the small building trembled for hours.

Somehow, I slept.

The next morning, I trekked to see my first kuru patient, Wanitaba. To each patient I brought a blanket and a bar of soap—a generic unwrapped waxy cake, colored a dull brown, a cross between Ivory and lye. These were comforts that the sick didn't possess and that the native healers couldn't provide.

When I arrived in her hamlet, a band of elders assembled. An old man stooped on the bare skin of his behind and lit a handmade bamboo pipe. A few leaves dangled around his waist, and around his neck he wore a string of white conch shells. Shells are highly valued currency because of their scarcity, imported hundreds of miles from the coast, bartered from one tribe to the next as they slowly ascended into the Highlands. Traditionally, trade was rare, transportation nil. One nearby tribe had no word in its vocabulary for what lay over the largest mountain on their horizon because no tribesman had ever been there. This culture was not outfitted for overnight travel. Their world was limited to what could be walked in a day.

With the elders assembled, I inquired about the patient, Wanitaba, and then constructed a family tree, finding out who else had died of kuru, which of these people had been eaten, and at which feasts the patient had been present.

Then, I ducked into a thatched hut to examine her. A quiet calm pervaded the cool darkness inside, interrupted only by the occasional crackle of a fire smoldering in the center. My eyes grew accustomed to the smoke, to the blackness, and to the vague, unfamiliar shapes of Stone Age paraphernalia suspended from the walls. I made out the form of the patient I had come to inspect, bundled up against the wall. I knelt down beside her. I thought her eyes flickered for a moment, though almost imperceptibly, as if to follow me. Her body shook and her head trembled because of her illness. I noticed that her eyes were still shining, although her body was preparing her for death. The family and villagers huddling around all knew her fate. They were there to mourn as much as to care for her. The house seemed a tomb of bamboo.

Though I had read countless textbooks and scientific articles about the disease and knew how to test for it on a physical examination with a cooperative patient, it was different with an actual case. She was too wasted for me to examine her fully. I was to learn about her by what the villagers taught me. They had seen countless cases of slow virus infections, far more than any hospital-based clinician in the West.

I took as detailed a history as I could. At first, Wanitaba had needed a stick to walk with, but she worsened and soon could no longer garden or perform daily tasks. Next, she lost the ability to stand, and spent the day sitting, eventually barely able to support her torso upright. Finally, a few weeks ago, her body had been laid here on the ground, quavering.

I placed my hand on her warm shoulder. I wished I could have passed on more than speechless reassurance. She did not speak my language nor I hers, and even if we had shared a tongue, I don't know whether she could have heard me. With that I got up to go.

Each day, I visited other patients reported to suffer from the disease. I performed neurological exams on them and documented which ones were truly infected with the disease and which merely had a bruised knee or a headache.

The data I collected from this region showed that in three different villages, two or more victims of the disease had been present together at only one or two feasts. In other words, clusters of patients had been infected simultaneously. These patients' exposures to the virus could be identified, and consequently the period of time the virus took to incubate in its victims' bodies could be measured. In two of these clusters of patients, the virus had simmered for twenty-five years, not affecting its hosts outwardly until less than one year before causing death. These were the longest incubation periods ever demonstrated for any known disease, and they substantiated Gajdusek's radical hypotheses about slow unconventional viruses. In two of the three villages, the patients died within months of each other. In one of the three villages, three young boys, relatives of one another, were exposed simultaneously. One died seven years later, and two died after twenty-five years. The incubation period could be identical but need not be. What the virus does for all these years remains unknown, but is important—recently with regard to AIDS as well.

While visiting this region, I met a leading medicine man, Satuma. He wore a battered, brown wide-brimmed hat. Articles of Western clothing were rare in this remote region. Hats were prized as decoration, and several men wore them—often old knit berets with pom-poms, or ski hats sent via missionaries from folks back in Nebraska. Satuma had managed to obtain an old Australian outback hat with a brim which was unraveling from the rest of the hat, and was held in place by a rusty safety pin, itself a unique item which he had fixed prominently in front as if it were a jeweled brooch. Like most men in the tribe, he occasionally donned traditional dress of leaves around his waist. His feet were bare.

My guide introduced us, and told him about me in their native tongue. Satuma greeted me warmly as a colleague. He proudly delineated his treatments and cures, reciting lists of cases—both successes and failures—which he stored in his head. His therapy for the disease was stringent—not to drink water or eat salt for a week and not to touch members of the opposite sex. Herbal medicines were also provided. Many of the panicked patients were cured, those whose symptoms I considered psychosomatic. Others progressed in their disease and began to tremble. All of his treatment failures were patients I had independently seen and diagnosed with the disease.

"Why are some patients dying despite treatment?" I inquired. His answer was simple. They hadn't followed his orders; they had drunk water, eaten salted food, and/or touched a spouse. To invoke the term doctors often use in explaining their treatment failures in Western hospitals, these patients were "noncompliant." There was only so much a doctor could do—in Papua New Guinea or in the United States.

But while I believed the disease was caused by a virus, Satuma and the Fore believed it was spread by sorcery. A tribesman cast spells on his enemies by stealing their belongings. Initially, a fragment of a skirt was thought necessary for the magic to succeed. More recently, after walls around hamlets were constructed to keep the sorcerers out, even a scrap of a potato peel was rumored to suffice. The booty was wrapped with leaves around a stone and buried in the ground as a malediction was uttered. The stone would shake, and when this happened, its victim was said to shake as well.

To ensure success, these bundles were said to have been buried recently in the dirt of newly engineered roads. Jeeps rumbling over the stones would more readily induce tremors in the victim.

The Fore scoured desperately for cures. They tried bloodletting, shooting bamboo arrows into patients' calves with special short bows.

The South Fore also copied what they perceived to be effective remedies from the North. The North Fore were closer to the Goroka Valley, where Westerners had penetrated earlier. The whites brought with them a revulsion toward cannibalism, and pressured the natives to abandon the custom on moral and religious grounds—not for health reasons, since Gajdusek had not yet linked kuru with cannibalism. The South Fore continued their mourning practices longer—often surreptitiously, risking arrests—still refusing to acknowledge any connection between their feasts and this disease.

In the early 1960s, while the epidemic raged, the North Fore began to hold mass meetings, called *kibung*, in which reputed sorcerers were asked to confess and repudiate their practices. Several did. But the disease continued. Over the next few years, the incidence of the disease decreased among the North Fore, coincident with the curtailing of cannibalism over the previous decade. When the South Fore observed the eradication of the disease among their neighbors, they concluded that the *kibungs* of several years earlier had been effective. The South Fore adopted this practice and held meetings. However, the disease continued unabated, as they had continued cannibalism longer than their northern neighbors. The *kibungs* constituted an attempt at cure that had been tried and found to be successful elsewhere. A parallel chain of logic pervades American medicine, where proposed medications are first investigated in clinical trials and then employed widely on patients. Claims made for the new drugs by eager pharmaceutical firms often turn out to have been exaggerated.

Both Westerners and Stone Agers thus want cures, need them, and believe they have them, citing objective evidence in support of their views, desperate for the opportunity to fight in some way against the onslaught of disease. Efficacy in New Guinea depends on the existence of psychosomatic cases, which may have been recognized, in part, to continue to prove that cures worked. They gave the Fore hope. There is a need for a cure, onto which families and patients can pin hope even as it flutters away. While Westerners look for diagnoses to explain suffering, the Fore seek cures.

The Fore asked why white men had not cured the disease, if they thought they knew what caused it. Westerners are aware that the process of developing effective medical treatment for a new disease can be slow. However, to the Papua New Guinean this question served as a rigorous evaluative criterion. In selecting between hypotheses, the correct theory is the one that leads to a cure, the one that works.

"Kuru is caused by a very small living organism," I explained to them, "much smaller than an insect."

"Can you show it to us?" they asked.

"It is too small to see with your eye and requires a special instrument to view it."

"Do you have any pictures?"

"None have been taken yet." The virus had not yet been isolated.

"What does it look like then?"

"Scientists aren't sure."

"Has anyone ever seen it?"

"It's not clear that anyone has."

"You white men don't make sense," they said and laughed. "We know that kuru is caused by kuru bundles, which we have seen." Unearthed bundles had been publicly displayed, supporting the belief that these parcels existed and had "caused" the illness.

"But the disease is decreasing," I pointed out, "because the traditional mourning feasts have been stopped, which used to spread the disease. Many small children had kuru in the past because they were present at these feasts. Small children are no longer dying of the disease. Over the past few years, the youngest children to die of it have been getting older." My audience wasn't impressed.

"That's because the sorcerers heard our pleas," they answered, "and stopped casting spells on young children. Sorcerers know better now. Children haven't made them mad." Statistics I cited had little meaning or impact. The members of this tribe had never read numerical charts or graphs. Nor did they systematically review the ages of patients. Every one of these adults had lost a parent or close relative to the disease. They knew people who still fell victim each year.

The logic of these tribesmen was impossible to refute without first persuading them that psychosomatic cases existed and that purported cures were only effective as placebos.

Satuma and I both looked for causes. A Western doctor re- assures, explaining suffering. But prognoses weren't important to the Fore. To one of my patients, I might declare, "This disease is infectious," or "It looks grim." Satuma couldn't say these things. In the West, a family is often helped by knowing death is inevitable. This pronouncement abets resignation, easing the transition of mourning. The Fore wailed loudly at the kuru funerals I attended, hoping for a reversal in this suspected man-made plague. Women chanted and cried in loud falsettos. They were outraged at the sorcerers in their midst.

The native healer offered more to the Fore than I did. He thought his cure worked, and his patients believed it. He had a cause that his patients accepted and he had reasons to explain away his failures. I had none of these.

Western medicine has many powerful drugs—antibiotics have saved countless lives. Insulin has helped millions of diabetics, although many have died anyway from not following medical advice and prescribed regimens. Patients with coro- nary artery disease will indulge in high-cholesterol diets, de- fying professional, high-cost instructions. Other diseases still lack cures. Our balance sheet reveals a mixed performance. For every magic bullet, there's a voodoo pin. As an intern, I had seen that a patient's beliefs affect his choice of, and motivation for, treatment. Rates of noncompliance are high even for drugs that have been proven in laboratories to work. Faith in the effectiveness of a remedy also exerts a strong influence on the therapy's success.

Fore patients had all consulted the local medicine man be- fore they saw me, and their families had often paid dearly in pigs, the main traditional currency, and cash, which had recently filtered into the villages. On a medical ward, patients are dying but continue to get patched up. Interns, I had learned, often temper diseases more than they can cure them.

Healers do not always cure. The Fore healer offered Wanitaba more than I did, and I gave more to my patient Charlotte Row than he ever could. Neither of us eradicated their disease. But I learned that healers do not have to cure to be sought and respected, as they are imbued with the belief that they understand an illness and can offer some comfort.

Diseases themselves are culturally framed. The Fore possessed their own diagnostic scheme, with the number of diseases they recognized increasing over the years of progressive Western contact. In the West, more weight is put on diagnosis, in part to relieve patients that "No, you don't have cancer, just the flu." Diagnoses also help determine treatment and prognoses. To the New Guinean, prognoses weren't important. The passage of time wasn't measured as in the West. A society that didn't traditionally register more than three days forward or backward isn't curious about questions of how many years were left, and how imminent was death. They aren't encumbered by wills and other papers that needed to be "gotten in order." Westerners follow controlled drug trials and know that for specific subsets of disease, different medications are more or less effective. Our diagnostic schemes have been influenced by the availability of cures. Because we have treatments for various kinds of illnesses, we conceive of different illnesses as separate disease entities. We subtype leukemias because treatments and prognoses vary. The distinction between a *Klebsiella* pneumonia and a pneumocystis pneumonia is important because they are treated with different medications. To the Fore, lacking antibiotics and microbiology laboratories to draw such distinctions, these different ailments would be lumped together and considered identical.

Despite the Western vision of its medicine as universally applicable, proven, and efficacious, healers seemed to be culturally bound. In the West, efficacy of treatment is believed to determine almost wholly why patients see doctors. But often doctors merely slow death, not stop it.

Once, while walking with my New Guinean guides on a dirt path at night beneath a full moon, luminous in a cloudless sky, I asked, "Do you know, we've sent people to walk on the moon?"

"Oh yeah," one answered nonchalantly as if recalling that fact to himself, as if it were most natural.

"Really. They walked on the surface of the moon up there," I insisted, pointing toward the distant disc of light. He nodded. This time, he gave me a polite little smile.

" 'Em straight," he said in pidgin, from the English, "them straight," or "that's right." He displayed neither curiosity nor surprise. He no doubt wondered how I could be concerned about something so far away and separated from my daily life.

As I stood in Charlotte's temperature-controlled hospital room during my internship, New Guinea seemed far off. Four years had passed. I had been taught the formal foundations of medical science but little about the human element, the human interaction. I didn't bring back the smells of "the bush," but I remembered that what was important about a doctor's work is not always the cure he offers but something else.

The fear with which I had begun internship had yielded to greater confidence as a physician. But my initial idealism about a doctor's powers had been tempered. I had thought that much of my New Guinea experience would be irrelevant, and that during internship, I would cure almost all of my patients. I was wrong. The limits of a doctor's efforts became apparent, as did the ranges of possible aid. I had learned to expect less, thereby reducing my disappointments. Much of what I did as an intern was medical hand-holding, making someone more comfortable as he or she waited to die. Satuma would have questioned much of my activity each day, as I spent tens of thousands of dollars—the yearly income of his entire tribe— sustaining an unconscious person for a few extra days or weeks.

Charlotte Row lay surrounded by a push-button phone, a television set, and a tinted glass window peering down on the city. She suffered from CJD, Wanitaba from kuru. Their maladies were closely related. But Wanitaba was cared for primarily by her family and a tribal healer. For Charlotte, a university-trained medical staff shouldered the burden.

Until more research is done, one wouldn't be helped any more than the other.